STAFF SUPPORT IN HEALTH CARE

STAFF SUPPORT
IN HEALTH CARE

David J. Stoter *AKC, JP*

*Manager of the Chaplaincy Department and Bereavement Centre,
Queen's Medical Centre, Nottingham*

**Blackwell
Science**

© 1997
Blackwell Science Ltd
Editorial Offices:
Osney Mead, Oxford OX2 0EL
25 John Street, London WC1N 2BL
23 Ainslie Place, Edinburgh EH3 6AJ
350 Main Street, Malden
  MA 02148 5018, USA
54 University Street, Carlton
  Victoria 3053, Australia

Other Editorial Offices:

Blackwell Wissenschafts-Verlag GmbH
Kurfürstendamm 57
10707 Berlin, Germany

Zehetnergasse 6
A-1140 Wien
Austria

First published 1997

Set in 10.5/13pt Sabon
by DP Photosetting, Aylesbury, Bucks
Printed and bound in Great Britain by
Hartnolls Ltd, Bodmin, Cornwall

The Blackwell Science logo is a trade mark of
Blackwell Science Ltd, registered at the United
Kingdom Trade Marks Registry

DISTRIBUTORS

Marston Book Services Ltd
PO Box 269
Abingdon
Oxon OX14 4YN
(*Orders:* Tel: 01235 465500
          Fax: 01235 465555)

USA
Blackwell Science, Inc.
Commerce Place
350 Main Street
Malden, MA 02148 5018
(*Orders:* Tel: 800 759 6102
                 617 388 8250
          Fax: 617 388 8255)

Canada
Copp Clark Professional
200 Adelaide Street, West, 3rd Floor
Toronto, Ontario M5H 1W7
(*Orders:* Tel: 416 597 1616
                 800 815 9417
          Fax: 416 597 1617)

Australia
Blackwell Science Pty Ltd
54 University Street
Carlton, Victoria 3053
(*Orders:* Tel: 03 9347 0300
          Fax: 03 9347 5001)

A catalogue record for this title is available
from the British Library

ISBN 0-632-04098-X

Library of Congress
Cataloging-in-Publication Data

Stoter, David J.
  Staff support in health care/David J. Stoter;
  foreword by Christine Hancock.
    p. cm.
  Includes bibliographical references and
  index.
  ISBN 0-632-04098-X
  1. Medical personnel–Counselling of.
  2. Medical personnel–Job stress.   3. Burn
  out (Psychology)–Prevention.   4. Employee
  assistance programs.   5. Employee morale.
  I. Title.
  RC451.4.M44S76   1997
  610.69–dc21   97–10863
                                            CIP

I dedicate this book with gratitude to my wife Moira, and to my children Mark and Claire; also to the many hundreds of friends in the health and caring professions with whom I have been privileged to work over the years.

Contents

Contents

Foreword

Since the pioneering work of Isobel Menzies in the 1960s, considerable attention has focused on the pain and the difficulties experienced by many health care workers. Sadly, the importance of providing a healthy, caring and supportive environment for staff working in the health services is too often ignored or overlooked until a crisis occurs.

This book makes the case for staff support at a time when the pressures on staff are greater than ever before. The expectations of patients and their families are higher, encouraged by Government initiatives such as the Patients' Charter, and by a society more attuned to their rights. At the same time, economic pressures are more acute, advances in medical technology bring new ethical dilemmas for staff, and the shift away from hospital-based care has led to a new working and caring culture.

There is, of course, no easy route to providing effective support. A holistic approach such as that advocated by this book allows us to learn from the biological and behavioural sciences, to consider the context in which care is given, and to make the best use of resources – both people and money – that are available. We can then encourage strategies which promote a properly caring and supportive environment for the provision of health care, wherever it takes place.

The economic value of this approach is beginning to be recognised through studies of large organisations in the USA and others, such as the Post Office, in the United Kingdom. Proper staff support makes sound business sense.

However, the principles outlined in *Staff Support in Health Care* and advocated by the National Association for Staff Support, can also be applied in smaller and more local contexts: the busy general practice; the residential care home; or the community team working with local authority social services.

The book is therefore a valuable resource for staff in the many situations where health and personal care are given. It does not shrink from addressing the many difficult questions which staff who give care – and those who manage the delivery of the service – face in a stringent economic climate and an organisational culture of change. It gives hope that we can adopt strategies which reduce stress and its costs, minimise the risk of complaints and enhance the quality of patient care.

Christine Hancock   BSc (Econ), RGN
General Secretary of the
Royal College of Nursing

Preface

'No man can reveal unto you aught but that which already lies half asleep in the dawning of your knowledge.

The teacher ... if he is indeed wise he does not bid you enter the house of his wisdom, but rather leads you to the threshold of your own mind'

Kahil Gibran: *The Prophet*

Introduction

Twenty years ago the hospital where I worked was developing pioneering research in the field of leukaemia. At that time the death of children receiving this treatment was particularly high, in some categories 97% of those involved. A new specialist unit was established to provide revolutionary treatment and special care for these children. I could see this was going to create a heavy burden for staff caring for these children. They would be constantly dealing with emotionally demanding situations, not only with the children's distressing conditions but also with distraught and bereaved parents and families.

Support for the staff was clearly going to be needed on a regular basis. A suggestion put forward to this effect was dismissed with the statement that 'all the staff in this unit have been especially chosen as professionals highly skilled and specially selected to pioneer this work. They will be able to cope admirably.'

Three months after it opened the unit was reaching breaking point. Staff sickness and absenteeism were so serious that the unit was relying heavily on agency staff. More than half the team had signalled their intention to move to another post and recruitment had become almost impossible. At this point I was invited to go in and provide support as a matter of urgency. I can still picture vividly the scene at that first meeting of staff in the unit. We used the ward sister's office, with staff from all disciplines using every available space, even sitting on the window sills, sharing chairs or sitting on the floor. They began to describe what the work was like, how awful the illness was for the children and their families, and revealing the emotional impact of those painful experiences on themselves.

One admitted to having nightmares, and others agreed. Some admitted problems with sleeping and eating patterns. Many felt unable to join in their usual social activities and some noticed that their family relationships were being disturbed. As their courage grew, so they began to realise that they were not alone in this, which brought a great sense of relief. They all felt 'we need help', and soon it became 'we can help each other'. Out of that meeting the first staff support group was formed, which I facilitated. Regular meetings took place in the same cramped office; they would not move from that room. Soon resignations were withdrawn, sickness rates fell below the norm experienced elsewhere and recruitment ceased to be a problem; in fact competition for posts grew. Before long, other sections of the hospital and in nearby locations began to ask for support groups. There were many lessons to be learned from this for management, for the team and for those offering support. We will explore the issues raised by this example later in the book.

I have long been convinced of the need for an *integrated response to need* to bring a change in the culture of care and identification of good patterns of staff care, which feed through into high quality patient care. I have been encouraged by preliminary research evidence supporting this conviction, indicating it is high time for a systematic approach throughout the service.

This book is an attempt to *look at staff needs* in this light and to suggest how staff care can be advanced in all sections of the caring professions. This cannot be viewed through simplistic responses, and the discussion draws heavily on personal experience, observation and research from a range of sources.

The nature of the subject

Many good books and well researched papers have been written in recent years on stress and its management. It is fashionable to say 'I am stressed out' as a statement of personal congratulation, but with no intention of doing anything about it. The statement is often used in relation to a family or work situation, without necessarily requiring any response or action from anyone.

This book attempts to stand back and take a good look across the range of perspectives on this subject which has accumulated over recent years. Holistic perspectives on matters related to health are important and relevant, with so many perspectives interrelated and interdependent. This approach helps to identify priorities, where resources are limited, in tackling the basic causes of stress and preventing unnecessary damage. It makes for better team work and helps individuals to feel more confident in what they can offer by taking personal responsibility and knowing what they are doing. There are many advantages. The subject is vast, so a disciplined approach is necessary to create a strategic policy that will achieve results.

How to use the book

This book is designed to serve a range of purposes and suit many readers at different stages of their careers. It concentrates on drawing out *principles* from current thinking and on using current *research* to throw light on some perspectives of the subject leading to appropriate action.

The text is presented in five sections, each divided into chapters dealing with a particular perspective. The book can be used as a reference text and sections or chapters can be read individually as aspects of the subject to be studied in their own right. There is a logical sequence to the text as the *process* of staff support is developed. This enables readers to use the book as a developmental study of the subject and a basis for course work and personal development.

The complex nature of the subject makes it essential to have an understanding of the principles involved in providing staff support if any provision is to achieve satisfactory results. For this reason the progression starts with an exploration of the nature of stress and traces the development of *knowledge* about it. Ways of identifying the *origins* of stressful pressures are explored, which is an important basis to an *understanding* of the subject. This foundation of understanding is essential for anyone wishing to make provision for a good staff support system.

This progressive approach is outlined in the following figure, which shows how the various aspects of staff support can be broken into smaller sections for ease of study and management, then how these aspects can be brought together in a practical way to formulate an informed and strategic plan of action right for a particular location.

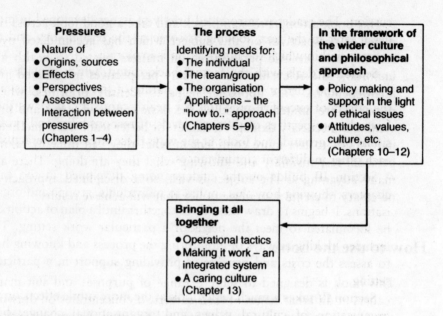

Progressive approach to setting up a staff support system.

The figure shows that staff support is more than a 'one-off' decision, but is an on-going process involving all staff in an organisation.

Examples drawn from professional and life experience are given wherever appropriate, to illustrate points. Exercises designed to help understanding and practical application appear at the end of each chapter. These are also questions useful for essay topics or for a focal topic in a discussion group. The wide range of references given provides material for further study or evidence as a foundation for action.

While it may appear that the book is designed for hospitals and the National Health Service, the basic principles introduced in the text are fundamental for any practitioner wherever they are based – in specialist areas, in the community, in general practice, in hospice care or in private medicine.

Progression through the book

In Section I the opening chapter offers a general introduction, relating staff support to quality care and defining the parameters of the discussion. The reader is introduced briefly to issues developed in more detail later in the text, looking at some of the terminology and the context within which the information is explored.

Section II deals with the factual background, which provides the evidence and current thought on the nature of stress, its origins, and the effects of excessive pressures for health care staff. It views these from the perspectives of different levels of responsibility and professional background, and looks at the ways these stressors interact with each other in different circumstances.

Section III builds on the understanding developed in the early chapters, showing how this applies to individuals, groups and organisations. It begins to draw these three together until a plan of action can be formulated to meet the needs of a particular work setting. This includes looking at ways of monitoring the process and knowing how to assess the costs and benefits of providing support in a particular setting.

Section IV takes a much wider look at the more subtle effects on the organisation of cultural values and organisational change, both internally and externally. Factors affecting society can bring accompanying insecurities and threats, all of which can add to pressures on individuals and organisations. This section also looks at pressures generated by some controversial ethical issues, and recognises the need for a constantly adaptive approach on the basis of a sound philosophy and a realistic policy.

Section V draws together the in-depth analysis of issues throughout the text into a synthesis, giving an overview of how the system can form an integrated or holistic approach to staff support, sifting out the priorities for action and recognising the interactions between them and how these affect the whole picture. All the principles involved can be used and adapted to any situation, leading to a highly effective and strategically planned support system.

Each reader will find something to help meet particular requirements, and hopefully will find new and creative ideas and suggestions, as well as gaining increased confidence through an overall understanding of the many complex issues involved in creating a realistic staff support system in a caring culture. This is not the nebulous 'soft option' it may seem; it is a very sophisticated approach which involves serious consideration of all the available evidence. It involves an intelligent use of resources and information to develop a good foundation that will outlast any changing organisational structures and cultural attitudes.

'Look with your understanding. Find out what you already know and you will see the way to fly'

Richard Bach: *Jonathan Livingstone Seagull*

David J. Stoter
October 1996

Acknowledgements

As always in writing and producing a book there are many people to thank for the enormous amount of help and encouragement given during the process.

My thanks go to Grace Owen for her advice and support in editing the manuscript and for the detailed work on referencing and indexing the book.

Thank you to Janet Morriss for her expertise in collating the material and preparing the disk for the printers, and to Kathryn Steady for her efficient work in preparing the typed manuscript.

Thanks also go to Griselda Campbell and her team for their encouragement and patience during the production process.

I would like to acknowledge the National Association for Staff Support, for the encouragement given by its members, and for giving me access to resource material and research papers from Central Office.

I would also like to acknowledge the following for permission to reproduce excerpts in this book:

Handy, C. (1995) *The Age of Unreason*. Arrow Business Books, Random House, London.

MSF (1995) *MSF Guide: Preventing Stress at Work* (Safety Information No. 40). MSF Health and Safety Office, Bishop's Stortford.

Quoist, M. (1992) *The Breath of Love*. Gill and Macmillan Publishers, Dublin.

Eliot, T.S. (1969) *Collected Poems 1909–1962*. Faber and Faber, London, and Harcourt Brace & Company, London.

Smith, A. (1976) Social Change. Addison Wesley Longman, Harlow.

Every effort has been made to contact copyright holders for permission to reproduce material published in this edition.

Every effort has been made to contact copyright holders for permission to reproduce material published in this edition.

Section I

The Process of Staff Support

Chapter 1

Staff Support – Quality Care

> 'Would you tell me please which way I ought to go from here?'
> 'That depends a good deal on where you want to get to,' said the Cat.
> 'I don't much care where –' said Alice.
> 'Then it doesn't matter which way you go' said the Cat.
> '– so long as I get *somewhere*,' added Alice as an explanation.
> 'Oh you're sure to do that,' said the Cat, 'if, you only walk long enough.'
>
> Lewis Carroll: *Alice's Adventures in Wonderland*

The ultimate purpose of good staff support is to ensure the highest possible standards of care for patients. These standards can only be delivered if there is also high quality staff care. Well integrated staff support practices, recognised and acceptable to all staff, are essential in any health care setting. The quality of care offered to patients is influenced considerably by the extent to which the carers themselves feel valued and cared for. This fact was first recognised by Revans (1962) and has since been demonstrated by many others (summarised by Hingley 1991).

Equipment in any intensive care unit is checked and serviced regularly in order to ensure reliability and effectiveness, as a patient's survival may depend on this. The same principles apply to the care of staff working in the caring services. The human resource is a vital and expensive item in the budget. Taking care of people is even more important than caring for machinery, and care of staff is vital in ensuring safe delivery of care for patients. To maintain high quality care, health care professionals need to be fit and healthy so that they can function at their best. Staff who are under pressure, stressed and overtired can make serious mistakes. If proper servicing of machinery and equipment is an indication of the importance attached to its functioning, it follows that staff care needs the same kind of recognition. Thus, good staff support is an indication of the value placed on the members of the workforce.

> The advertising section of a recent health care journal contained nine different advertisements for a 'support manager' or a 'support officer' and the job description included the words 'to care for and service IT equipment'. No advertisement was found, in that or several other journals, for a post for a support manager for staff care, or indeed for any post with that kind of job description. Advertisements for personnel officers usually described the job as 'managing, training or deploying staff', with no mention of staff care.

Issues involved with staff support

A necessity – or luxury?

Good staff support is not an optional extra. There is ample evidence that failure to provide support is costly, especially where conditions are stressful. Such failure may, in financial terms, amount to as much as 10% of the organisation's total expenditure (Cooper *et al.* 1990). In human terms, it can cause untold misery through stress-related illness, together with difficult team relationships, organisational dysfunction and resentment. There is growing evidence of the preventive value of good staff support practices. Although quantifiable evaluation is difficult, any costs involved are far outweighed by the benefits to staff, patients and the organisation (Cox 1993).

The many facets of stress

There are many ways of defining stress. The *Concise Oxford Dictionary* has at least five definitions. The variations are explored in the next chapter. What is generally described as 'stress' is an inevitable and essential component of normal living. A certain amount of stress is essential to all areas of life and types of activity (Montague 1979). Living involves adapting to circumstances surrounding us every day, in ordinary, everyday events as well as moments of crisis. It is a process which is essentially creative, but when stimulus and response do not balance there can be damaging effects on the individual, especially when this builds up over a long period.

The damaging effects of this unbalanced response to stress are well known (Cooper 1988; Hingley & Marks 1991; NASS 1992a). In addition to physical or emotional damage to the individual, Cox *et al.* (1990) notes a number of 'organisational effects' as he outlines the damage to an organisation in terms of poor productivity and industrial relations and increased absenteeism.

There are many examples of the appropriate use of stress in creative situations, such as the actor preparing off-stage for a leading role, or the artist or writer under pressure to produce a piece of work. An athlete demonstrates several elements of the creative use of stress generated by the pressure to achieve success and support the team. The same is true in other aspects of life. However, when stress causes an unbalanced response, perhaps due to frustration or fear of failure, the effects become negative and harmful. *Balance* is the important factor; when there is an imbalance between positive and negative pressures, a situation becomes out of control. Control is retained where the balance is maintained. These are fundamental factors when considering the value of staff support.

Staff relationships

The quality of relationships between staff is important in maintaining staff morale. People differ in the way they relate to others. Some people perform best in a team, while others are at their best when working alone. Faced with the same situation, some people will be disabled by challenges which diminish their capacity to perform, while others will thrive and produce an enhanced response. This factor is crucial in the selection of staff and contributes to good staff support. This is why it is so important, when choosing a person for a particular job, to identify someone who will be able to work creatively within the situation. One problem in health care services has been the assumption that good clinical skills and length of service make a person suitable for leadership or management.

In situations of immediate challenge, the qualities needed are found in staff who can respond and adapt swiftly and take responsibility for decision making. There are other situations which demand a longer, cooler look at events and therefore require different skills.

We need to know ways to recognise and identify the stress which

- is inherent in a situation;
- is created by the response of one or more people;
- is destructive;
- is creative;
- is generated by the response to the situation;
- could be minimised or eradicated.

These points illustrate some of the many facets of stress which are related to staff support. These and many others should be acknowledged, and provision to meet these needs should be built into the system.

The philosophy of care

A philosophy of care should be the prevailing attitude permeating through every level of the services within an organisation. People who give care need to be able to receive care themselves. They too have human needs which must be recognised and acknowledged. Provision for these needs should be built into the system and made available at all times to everyone in the organisation. Often there can be 'double standards'. There has been a traditional ethos among health carers that failure to cope with pressures alone and under all circumstances is a sign of failure or weakness, and to an extent this attitude still prevails in some organisations.

There is a tendency to see ourselves as either 'carers or 'being cared for', while in current thinking the caring relationship involves the concept of 'partnership' between patients, relatives and professionals. There is, however, evidence that this approach is not yet widely established, although it is much talked about (Owen 1989; Bayntum-Lees 1992; Stoter 1995a). Where the giving and receiving of care and support for staff is seen to imply weakness and failure, this can have a profound impact on the nature of care and support given to patients and relatives, inhibiting the partnership philosophy and causing paternalistic and maternalistic care giving.

Quality care

Quality care for patients and families depends heavily on the staff who deliver that care and on the kind of environment created; any anxiety is readily passed on to patients and others. Stressed staff create a stressful atmosphere, which may lead to a stressful response from patients and their families. Points to consider are:

- Relationships between staff care and patient care
- What happens when stress ceases to be creative
- How this affects colleagues and patients.

There is evidence to show a direct relationship between staff care and patient care. Recovery and turnover rates of patients are also affected

(Revans 1990; Booth 1995). It is uncomfortable being with those who are very stressed and is not conducive to building up a relationship of trust between the care giver, the patient and the family.

When equilibrium is lost and pressures become excessive, responses become negative in their effect and move away from an enhanced response to an inhibitive response. The care giver's ability to identify accurately the needs of patients and relatives diminishes, as does the ability to select the right options of care, and so the whole quality of care is diminished. This can have a 'downward spiral' effect on group morale.

Those who are affected by the negative aspects of stress may become aggressive to those around them and can become brusque, with distressing effects on patients and relatives.

A young woman was visiting her father who had been admitted to the accident and emergency department of a large hospital. He had had a suspected heart attack. Over several weeks he was making a steady recovery and had been transferred between various wards and departments for emergency care, diagnosis, treatment and rehabilitation – four different care situations altogether. His lively accounts of the kind of care he was receiving intrigued his daughter.

After several weeks he was a veteran and his observations became astute and more sophisticated and critical. He summed up his views one day, by saying:

'You know, where the staff team, doctors, nurses and all the others are respected, valued and consulted, they care for each other. The patients get better care and treatment. The staff explain things, they talk to us and we get better more quickly because we are confident.' He noticed also that difficult patients became co-operative and relatives were less pressurised. He left some wards feeling they were happier places than others. 'You get better more quickly and feel good,' was his final observation to his daughter.

Staff support – what it involves

When we accept that staff support must be addressed and is not just an optional extra, for good patient care and efficient service, the next question to consider is the nature of the staff support. This is where many different interpretations exist, as shown by the following example.

Conference participants were invited to write a brief definition of staff support as they understood it. These responses show the wide variation of perceptions.

Staff support is:

- about an organisation having mechanisms in place to help staff who may be experiencing unwanted stress
- not only to be reactive but proactive
- genuine care at *all* levels, which encourages those in great and small posts of responsibility to feel equally important
- enabling people to be fully and creatively present in the work they do
- a collection of safety nets by which providers of services can feel held, regarded and valued
- about empowering and enabling individuals to care more effectively for themselves and for others
- providing the same sort of health service for staff as one would for patients
- about caring for staff – understanding their needs – being available on the spot – listening – sharing in problems – ensuring people know where they can find and use services which can help in the longer term – ensuring those services are available
- mechanisms that help to create an environment of care whereby individuals are enabled or empowered to receive and give care.

The caring culture

To provide a general ethos of staff care through staff support, a broad approach is essential as it involves much more than setting up a few systems or services. Setting up a counselling service or extending the occupational health department will be important specific services to consider, but unless these are backed up by a range of accessible services, an informed communication system and staff willing to use them, they can be expensive investments with little return.

Good staff support involves primarily the creation of a caring and supportive working environment and a 'culture which is an integral part of every institutional setting and not just a service brought in when other things break down' (Stoter 1991). Staff support should be seen as a preventive service providing support at the point of need; without this any existing services can at times become overloaded and unmanageable.

There are three main aspects to consider when setting up a good support system and these will be explored throughout the book:

- We need to start with ourselves and take some responsibility (at all levels within the organisation) for our own personal welfare and environment
- We then move on to caring for one another in the wider teams or groups
- We need to consider the organisational setting, looking at the wider culture and the services available.

Effecting change

Some relevant issues have been introduced briefly in this chapter, and the next few chapters explore in more depth the complex nature of challenges faced by health care staff. It will then be possible to identify the pressures and the role of staff support in reducing their effect. This in-depth approach may seem daunting especially if urgent solutions are being demanded of staff who are often asked to produce ideas for staff support systems at short notice, so finding themselves in a position where they want to solve a problem now but there are no short cuts. If they cannot offer a quick solution they become so devastated that they cease to function well, feel overwhelmed by the situation and slip into a downward spiral approach which affects those around them, so adding to the pressures.

Anyone planning a journey on an unfamiliar route will do well to have a look at the map to sort out the best routes. They will recognise the limitations of their transport and the resources available; a clear vision of the possibilities and solutions will facilitate planning ahead, with greater assurance of achieving something. This approach can be applied to the process of setting up a staff care service.

A clear example of this is seen in the life of Nelson Mandela who took over 30 years to achieve his goal of a peaceful revolution. In the early years he was faced with two options. Many of his followers would have liked him to arm and go for open rebellion, which would almost certainly have led to bloodshed and a massacre, which would have defeated the objectives and destroyed the opportunity for all time. Instead, he went for the grand gesture of inaction and during the waiting period he was all the time feeding

(Contd)

> information into the minds of others, establishing communications, writing articles for the press, making sure the world could see the problems, and seeking out good contacts. People began to see that they could not allow the injustices to go on for ever; the inequalities must be addressed or there would inevitably be bloodshed and much more. As fear mounted this began to get through to those in power who were in a position to effect change, and eventually there came a white president who realised he might be the last. He could see the inevitable was on its way and effected change. All this needed endless patience, waiting and taking one step at a time until achievement was in sight. Any other route could have led to destruction and disaster.

Some readers may be asking, 'How on earth am I going to achieve anything? Where do we start? How can I begin?'. It may be that everything in the workplace is not as we would wish; colleagues and managers are not as we would like them to be. We may feel out of tune with government policy and with professional practice. For many of us this is reality and where we have to start. As we begin to broaden our perspectives it may be possible to see areas where change is possible. There are others who share our vision, so it may be possible to start a chain reaction from a small local initiative which gathers popularity and brings encouragement as it grows.

It is possible to feed ideas into minds to bring about change. As people see the benefits of changes they will be won over, and this will influence those who have the power to effect wider changes in the organisation. Our vision of what creates a just society and what is right for staff, to enable them to become valued and respected, must be matched by confidence that changes will happen as people recognise their worth, and so there will be results. There are effective ways of achieving these ideals through working with management to improve the environment. It is possible to persuade colleagues, who are themselves in positions of influence with others, that improvements can be effected, by using new evidence and convincing results. Ideas will eventually permeate the power base and the whole organisation. Pioneers, wherever they work in the organisation, need encouragement and support. Small changes, wherever they occur, are important and these small changes gain a momentum and build up to infiltrate the wider environment in the workplace. This affects the organisation as a whole, so creating a caring culture. All of this needs time, as we saw in Nelson Mandela's experience. It needs to be based on such research findings and evidence as are available, and can be used in conjunction with local evaluation of needs and assessments of priorities.

Changes are best achieved when people are aware of the possibilities ahead, are informed about the areas where change is possible, and are willing to take opportunities as they occur. Successful outcomes are achieved when staff are able to participate and are kept informed when a policy is being decided. Little will be achieved without this involvement, if a new staff care system or new services are to be used. To embark on a programme of total reform at once may not be feasible, but most staff will find it possible to select some local initiatives they can begin to develop. They may learn to recognise areas where change can be effected and so the whole process will gain momentum, with staff informed and prepared to transform vision into reality. This book will be exploring many of those initiatives, and ways in which all staff can be involved and can benefit by changes in their workplace.

'A tree as big around as you can reach, starts with a small seed; a thousand mile journey starts with one step'

Benjamin Hoff: *The Tao of Pooh*

Key points

(1) Quality staff support ensures quality patient care.
(2) Stress is a feature of all normal life and activity.
(3) Stress can be creative, but when it gets out of balance it can have destructive effects.
(4) Staff support has many different interpretations, and definitions range widely.
(5) Staff support includes a range of issues to be considered.

Exercises

(1.1) Write down *your* description of staff support.
(1.2) What aspects of staff support are evident in your workplace? Keep your response for reference later.

Section II

Pressures and Responses

Chapter 2

Pressures Identified – Knowing the Sources

The identification of pressures on staff is a complex process. It can be an easy option to state the popular, known causes of the damaging effects of stress which are often cited by the media and press. These are misleading to those attempting to find ways of coping with the pressures. There is a tendency to overlook the positive aspect of stress, which is creative and energising. A basic framework for assessment is useful to ensure confidence in tackling the real issues and in making an efficient use of resources. It is also helpful to explore the issues from several different perspectives, and to make an accurate diagnosis of the *local* situation to ensure the best remedies are found and applied.

The presence of excessive and stressful pressures is most frequently recognised by their effects on individuals, groups and wider organisations, and inevitably recognition must precede any attempt to identify the sources. To carry through this identification and discover the causes with any accuracy, it is essential to have an informed awareness of the nature of the effects. Many simplistic assumptions abound in the press and media, when the whole process is in fact complex with many interrelated variables. There are a number of useful models available taking different perspectives on the subject, although many deal with the more damaging and negative aspects of stress and ignore the creative aspects. It is useful for the reader to be familiar with some of these models in order to make an informed diagnosis of any situation. No one model provides a complete blueprint for action in all situations, but many can be used as a framework for understanding a situation and seeing it from different perspectives.

This chapter considers some models which can be particularly useful for health care workers when attempting an assessment. There is one simple basic framework which can be adapted for most of the perspectives explored in this text, as suggested by Biley's classification (Biley 1989). He states that pressures can be identified in three different ways:

(1) *Intrapersonal* or those concerning forces arising from within the individual
(2) *Interpersonal* or those forces occurring between individuals
(3) *Extrapersonal* meaning those forces exerted from outside the individual.

These categories offer a framework for formulating coping strategies. They can be used in formulating plans for a support system, as described by many practitioners and authors, so this simple classification is basic to many of the following discussions.

Identification of a stressful workplace

For all health care workers, whether in a hospital unit or community setting, the workplace is bound to be pressured. By the nature of the occupation there will be emergencies and life threatening events, frequent moments of dealing with suffering and distressed individuals, and often death. There is also an expectation by professionals that there can be a satisfactory provision of total health care. These expectations are fuelled by the ever increasing growth of knowledge, expertise and technology and the range of drugs available. There is also the increased understanding and awareness by the public at large of what can be achieved. Radio, television, the press and popular literature allow people to see at firsthand the range of possibilities open to them.

Expectations are also influenced by the prevailing *cultural attitudes* of the day, particularly the 'them and us' approach referred to in the previous chapter. This attitude is not peculiar to health services, but exists throughout industry and other professions and creates considerable communication difficulties between management and staff. In a study by Traynor & Wade (1994) it was noted that many community nurses were saying they would like to 'go back to the good old days when the matron was in charge, compared with present management arrangements'. In fact those nurses could not have been old enough to have experienced the 'matrons' system and they were making assumptions on the basis of hearsay, so strong was the conviction that all management is 'bad'.

Further impetus is given to these expectations of a 'perfect provision of care' by the Department of Health's Patients' Charter. This lays down standards but implies these standards are to be expected. It encourages complaints where the ideals are not reached. For someone who has entered the caring professions mainly from a desire to care for others, there are many frustrations, and staff feel unfulfilled if they are unable to meet the standards as set out.

Carers and cared for

There is a tradition in the caring professions, which still influences attitudes, that carers who admit to fears of being 'unable to cope' show signs of weakness and unsuitability for the job. However, many of those who enter these professions are people of great sensitivity (Johnson 1991), a characteristic most desirable for delivery of quality care, but they are therefore vulnerable to the painful effects of suffering. This does not mean they are not suitable for the work they do, but it highlights the fact that their needs should be recognised and provision should be made for them. This useful quality can then be fully developed as a contribution to a caring professional practice. The traditional attitude mentioned above arises from the tendency for professionals to see themselves as 'care givers' and not 'care receivers', thus failing to accept that they too are human with needs that require recognition and attention. There is a tendency to fail to care for themselves adequately or take 'time out', so fatigue builds up as they fight against internal pressures. Fatigue decreases their ability to think clearly and evaluate situations accurately, and may lead to accidents and mistakes.

There are therefore several areas to consider when identifying the pressures that are inherent in the job, and these present conflicting demands:

• Attempts to maintain standards from past traditions in a changing scenario
• The expectations of patients and public
• Demands from government agents and management
• The carers' personal expectations of being able to deliver a high level of care at all times
• Traditional and cultural attitudes that may hinder good communications
• Lack of awareness and understanding of personal and colleagues' needs
• Inability to acknowledge the effects of pressures.

These expectations are intensified by the feeling of being undervalued and not respected by the government, the public at large and the institution. This leads to a lowering of self esteem as a sense of self worth is lost.

Identifying pressures at different levels and locations

The pressures outlined in previous paragraphs can affect all staff at all levels and in all professions, but the effects may be experienced and interpreted in different ways, both positively and negatively. It is important to recognise this as it calls for a range of constructive and preventive measures and an imaginative provision of staff support measures which will differ according to local circumstances.

People who *give care* need to be able to *receive care* if they are to be effective carers, hence the importance of starting with ourselves in looking at the various pressures we experience. This involves being able to *understand ourselves* and our reasons for responding as we do, and having a developing self awareness. People respond differently to situations according to personal characteristics, expectations and experiences. Experiences in early life shape expectations and personalities and make each of us a unique person. Environmental experiences in early life have considerable influence, and although there are several different schools of thought on this aspect, it is clear that the effect of painful experiences does shape our responses to stressful situations (Foss 1963; Rutter 1972; Storr 1981) A useful guide for employers published by the Health and Safety Executive (HSE 1990) acknowledges that:

> 'An existing challenge to one person may be a daunting task to another ... Much may also depend on the pressures which people are experiencing outside their work in their home and personal lives, bereavement, family sickness or worry ...'

Self acceptance and self knowledge

One important aspect fundamental to any analysis of stress in the workplace is recognition of the effects of stress, as seen in the response of individuals or teams. Recognition includes more than simply identifying the visible effects at any one time. It includes an acceptance that each one of us is vulnerable to an imbalance of excessive stress but our individual responses vary with our personalities or circumstances. Therefore *acceptance* is required to acknowledge that:

- Anyone can be affected given certain circumstances
- The ability to recognise the early signs and symptoms of harmful effects both in ourselves and in others is important
- An awareness of individual strengths as well as vulnerabilities is necessary
- Recognition and acceptance go together with an understanding of the way people respond
- Self knowledge and recognition of our own likely response is a good place to start.

At a workshop on stress management for health care staff the participants were invited in small groups to identify their own responses to stressful situations. It was surprising to hear a number of people say they did not show any signs of excessive stress and felt it showed a weakness to do this. As the discussion progressed, they were all able to begin to recognise and accept their own responses.

Recognition of the effects of stress

Many health care staff are familiar with signs and symptoms of excessive stress but they are unaware when these become damaging for them, unless they know their own likely responses. It is important for them to identify when the situation is beginning to have a negative impact and to recognise that they are moving into a negative cycle. The creative side of stress enhances and gives an edge to performances; it creates incentives and the ability to act and respond accurately and quickly to demands of life and work responsibilities. It gives a 'buzz' or a sense of wellbeing, of self worth and value with a purpose and challenge ahead. It stimulates creativity which extends to all aspects of life giving a sense of energy to home and family life as well as work situations, which generally makes a person look, sound and feel alive. There is a sense of being on top of things whatever happens, a feeling of being in control and in command with spare capacity. Meutz (1995) refers to the Health Education Authority classification which talks about constructive and positive stress, and destructive stress or the negative aspects (Health at Work in the NHS 1995a). The negative side is the opposite of the positive side and is brought about by an imbalance between the stimulus and response. At a personal level *early signs* may vary between individuals. These often start with:

- Disturbed sleep patterns with work activity not being up to usual performance standards
- A sense of being rushed, of work unfinished or incomplete and perhaps therefore not satisfying
- Things tending to take longer than usual
- A sense of difficulty in starting on a course of action
- Appearances may suffer with personal hygiene or dress becoming careless
- A strained look, with reactions such as irritability in company betraying pressure.

At this stage it is important to recognise both the positive and negative aspects of stress and to remember that both aspects have to be examined separately and responded to.

Negative responses to stressful situations

In addition to the signs listed above, as time goes by there are more serious effects. Social life may be affected, and there is increased irritability, short temper or sharpness, and misinterpretation of situations and instructions:

- Lack of interest in external activities
- Feelings of being too tired to join in usual relaxation, to go out with friends or family, or to go for a walk
- Carelessness over food, with meals missed which may lead to health problems, also loss or gain in weight. The problems escalate as the pressures build up, creating a downward spiral
- Work tends to become less satisfying and others are blamed for any failures in performance
- In particular there is increasing tendency to blame the employers and organisation, and to find excuses for any shortcomings
- At this stage anger and resentment build up internally and block the way for positive responses.

All this begins to affect the individual's health and work performance and so the ripples begin to extend to others in the team and to affect productivity and the organisation as a whole.

The important point is that recognition of signs at these early stages is essential if the process is to be checked or reversed before it does real damage to all concerned. Each of us can learn to identify our own ways of responding and to recognise the negative signs, which may start with disturbed sleep or irritability and feeling rushed. Some of us have a particularly significant response, like waking up in the night and checking to make sure we have not brought the keys of the drug cupboard home with us. We may be familiar with the urge to ring back to the ward and check that a certain treatment has been given, or the need to ensure the car has been locked. Others may have experienced driving into work and not registering passing through a particular place, and so feeling disorientated. Some have even been known to park the car at the wrong destination or arrive at the office and realise it was their day off. These examples are not unusual.

Effects on the health of the individual

It is important to recognise the build-up described above, and where possible to intervene and take appropriate action. If these early signs are ignored they are likely to have more damaging long term effects on health and result in any of the illnesses so frequently recognised as stress related and described by Cooper (1988) and Cooper and Smith (1986). The continuation of stress at these levels eventually damages the immune system (White 1990) and leaves the body vulnerable to more serious illnesses, including:

- Hypertension
- Migraine
- Pruritis
- Constipation or colitis
- Nervous dyspepsia
- Skin disorders
- Back problems

- Coronary thrombosis
- Asthma, hay fever and other allergies
- Peptic ulcers
- Rheumatoid arthritis
- Diabetes
- Depression.

This can also have an effect on the team, on their morale and performance levels. Once the negative effects begin to build up, their impact becomes even greater as a downward spiral increases the pressures and reinforces the tendency to negativism. This leads to a build-up of aggression, exaggeration of feelings of being undervalued, and hinders good communications.

Long term effects

Long term exposure to unrecognised or untreated stress results in wider effects as the ripples extend beyond the team into personal and family relationships. These pressures may lead to marital problems and social isolation, and in turn are reflected in increased sickness and absenteeism. This may lead to loss of job prospects and impaired work performance and productivity, as decision making becomes affected. There are further effects on industrial relations and accident rates which have significant implications for health care staff, with the possibility of serious drug errors, effects on the quality of patient care and turnover, and ultimately resulting in increased costs to the organisation (NASS 1992a; Cox 1993; Owen 1993). Other effects follow in terms of lowering of production, poor quality care, reduced performance levels and loss of team morale. (For a detailed discussion on this see Cartwright and Cooper 1994).

Pressures in different working situations

Sources of pressures will be recognised by similar negative effects on individuals, team performance and organisational operations, wherever they occur and at whatever level. For example, in the community they may originate within the primary care team or between hospital and community staff or social services. For community staff there may be strained relationships between the professionals and the local community or voluntary services. There may be different standards of care provision or failure to communicate through misunderstanding of jargon used. Feelings of isolation from the main activity may also play a part, especially where communications are lacking and staff feel remote from the centre. They may feel undervalued in the sense that they are underfunded and tend to get patients returned home with little support at a time when more active care is needed.

Another source of pressure can be found within the multidisciplinary team. Different professionals may well have different agendas or objectives to achieve. There could well be difficulties in trying to define a common definition of need, arising perhaps from the fact that a particular patient is cared for in different parts of the organisation, producing conflict in the timing of different parts of the treatment or rehabilitation programme. One source of tension may occur between professionals or treatment centres when there is a sense of rivalry for supremacy or leadership in the care programme. For example, there are situations where professionals regard themselves as practitioners in their own right, whereas others may feel they should only follow the requests that come from the medical team. There are different interpretations of language even between teams of the same professionals. A few years ago it was observed that there were up to twenty different interpretations on one ward of the doctor's instruction 'up and about'. This caused misunderstanding, errors and eventually tensions between staff. For example, some patients were allowed to sit out for one hour, some to walk to the bathroom, while others were allowed to stay up for 12 hours or even go home!

Other sources of pressure are found in the wider aspects of society and cultural groups, and these will be referred to later in the book.

The positive effects of pressures

Recognition of the *positive value* of stress is vital as it provides the ability to break into the vicious circle of negative effects by strengthening the positive ones and so redressing imbalance. The health care service today is a tough demanding environment where there are limited resources, and in this scenario staff can feel doomed to failure in achieving targets before they start. This attitude is perpetuated by the negative reporting in the media, and public demands for more and better services. Rarely is attention paid to the successes and examples of good care.

Fortunately there is plenty of evidence that some of the highest achievers and performers are often people who relish a challenging background of this kind, and find fulfilment in being able to achieve results through being creative and innovative. They are prepared to set achievable goals, to harness their own energy and that of others, and to recognise small achievements along the way. They find satisfaction in dealing with limited resources, finding alternatives and overcoming the problems, and find crisis situations stimulating. Examples of this attitude can be seen throughout history, where some new innovations and good ideas have been brought to fruition in times of war or deprivation. As Orson Welles pointed out, during the Borgia reign, Italy had 30 years of bloodshed and terror and produced the Renaissance, Leonardo and Michaelangelo. Switzerland had five hundred years of democracy and peace and produced the cuckoo clock.

> Examples can be seen in industry and commerce where innovative inventions have resulted from situations of overcoming limited resources. It may be that unreasonable shortages exist and therefore create unreasonable stress, but these resource limitations can be alleviated by proper
>
> *(Contd)*

allocation and planning ahead. Alternatively, a kind of bandwagon effect occurs where people reach and pass a certain point in their own stress response and their ability to think and plan ahead disappears. The guilt factor comes into play and they cannot say, 'If you expect this course of action with these resources from me I will fail'. Instead they may persist in working longer hours, which appears to be an easy way out of a situation. They then become tired and the harmful effects of excessive stress appear and they become ineffective. This builds up until the downward spiral of stress accumulates and they are no longer able to respond.

It is possible to hold together both the demands and limitations even within such unreasonable limits where a bandwagon effect has occurred. It is not always true that resources are limited, but to say this tends to be an easy way out of a situation. A balancing act has to be achieved of recognising the difficult factors and knowing that beyond a certain point it is impossible to deliver what is asked. Where the person is competent and confident of what they are doing they are able to address that situation and say, 'I cannot deliver what you ask within the remit you have given me. I can either deliver part of the remit, or if you allocate additional resources I will deliver the whole assignment effectively.'

In operating theatres we see an example of staff working within certain limits of hours, where cold surgery is concerned. Once those hours are filled, further cold surgery is cancelled. This is a way of limiting resources and overcoming a difficult situation. Alternatively they may say, 'Because resources are limited certain treatments are not available at present.'

This is one way of responding to the provision of a *safe* service, where resources are limited. It takes considerable strength of mind to make this kind of stand as many will be critical of postponing long awaited surgery. There are some who may argue: 'The important point in this situation is what you do with the resources you have'.

Another way of looking at response to lack of resources was experienced during the war years, when shortages generated new ideas which have persisted long after shortage ceased to be a problem. Some ideas stimulated new and creative inventions still in use. Food rationing prevailed and many cooks could make a meal from almost nothing because they had almost nothing to do it with, and everyone learnt a hundred different ways of preparing potatoes!

Someone who has not previously lived through a war can still adapt and learn to make do, as we have seen in recent events in Bosnia.

If this book is to achieve anything, it must inspire people to find a balance between the positive and negative sides of stress, so finding a way through to the creative aspects and breaking into the downward cycle of negative stress by enhancing the positive factors. We need to capture the individual's imagination, using their gifts and skills and welding them together in teamwork and eventually into the whole institution, in the context of trusting relationships. One point to which management must work is for each individual to have a common focus on creating the same environment of personal positivity within the team. It is about setting up a healthy and creative environment for patients and family. For example, industry and commerce have to attract customers, and managements have introduced ways of creating a sense of shared ownership in the business, which involves employees in sharing ideas and being asked to take a positive stance in the running of the business.

This is an essential point to grasp as we proceed to examine some of the current models for understanding stress. Inevitably some models are limited or only relevant to the particular situations under discussion. But it is important to be aware that a model is like a snapshot. In real life there are many variables interacting at any one time, and the overall picture is never static or one dimensional; there is always change, movement and interaction between the components.

Understanding stress

Before attempting to set up any support system it is essential to assess the situation and identify the sources of the pressures and the nature of their effects. As already mentioned, there are many variables to consider and any search for a simple approach through stress inventories of a general nature is unlikely to identify the real problem areas. There are a number of models, ranging from the very simple to the sophisticated, which can help us to understand the nature of the particular situation under review.

There are many good studies on the *nature and origins* of stress and how it affects different occupations. Each writer selects a particular approach and model that suits their purpose and so may not give a general view. Readers would be advised to become familiar with various approaches, because when viewed together they give an overall picture which can be useful in selecting the different perspectives needed for a particular assessment. A well known model related to organisational stress is put forward by Cooper *et al.* (1988).

Familiarity with these models and an understanding of the various approaches can bring a much more accurate perspective on the scenario to be assessed, and can help us to isolate the most vulnerable areas which need special consideration at once and to identify those where a longer term approach is adequate.

Approaches to understanding stress

Cushway (1995) offers a comprehensive discussion on the different perspectives on stress, which is helpful in giving an overall view. Difficulty in establishing a clear and meaningful definition of stress does give problems for researchers and practitioners who try to trace the origins of stress. A simple model which helps is the stimulus model (Payne & Firth-Cozens 1987) which emphasises the importance of the environment in relation to the individual's psychological response in order to help them to cope with environmental pressures. As Cox (1978) points out, this model does not allow for individual differences in response to similar situations.

One of the earliest models was Selye's response model (Selye 1950) where he sees stress as an internal response to external stressors, the dependent component being the stress shown by the individual under pressure. He identified the GAS (General Adaptation Syndrome), a model which Cushway points out is useful for those using a medical/ physiological concept, but is less popular with students of the organisational approach (Cushway 1995), and tends to avoid the psychological issues and stimuli.

A theoretical model currently favoured and combining the above two approaches presents an interactional approach. It considers the environmental and individual responses and the interaction between them, and is sometimes known as the *transactional model* (Lazarus & Folkman 1984). This model demonstrates a more realistic approach to the nature of stress. It points out that the negative effects (and most of the models do concentrate on the negative aspects) only arise when external demand exceeds the capacity of the recipient to respond and deal with it, and there is also a time variable involved before effects are apparent. This model does recognise more effectively the importance of the *individual aspects* of response, and the complexity of stress. Cushway points out these are the very aspects which are so difficult to measure or monitor accurately, and highlights the dynamic nature of the process. Harris (1991) suggests that this model may not adequately show the ways individuals respond, and so may give false identification of the common stressors in occupational settings. Readers may find it helpful to refer to some of these studies for detailed analyses.

None of these models is considered to give the whole picture of the origins of stress, neither can they give much help in deciding on the most appropriate coping mechanisms. Hingley and Marks (1991) conclude that this does not mean useful information cannot be gained from monitoring and attempting to evaluate outcomes. Cushway's article covers a range of issues basic to this subject and examines some methods of appraisal which we shall consider later.

One model, presented by Moss as a NASS conference paper (Moss 1995), includes the significance of personal factors as well as organisational aspects. It shows how organisational stress can affect the home and family situation and is then reflected back to the organisation.

Other approaches often cited include organisational models which tend to relate particularly to the workplace (Cooper 1988, 1995). These models are useful for studying certain aspects of a complex situation, which involve many dynamic interactive processes. Each model gives an insight into a particular approach. Such separate approaches are essential to enable research to be carried out in a specific area. Examples are given in Figs 2.1 and 2.2, but for a comprehensive picture an integrated model is needed, such as that in Fig. 2.3.

The identification of the origins of pressures is not simple. The media may seize upon what appear to be major issues, such as staff shortages, low pay or long hours, but if these were removed other pressures could appear. This complexity may be one of the reasons why some attempts to counteract negative effects seem to achieve little, and results are difficult to assess. It may also be why there sometimes appears to be little attempt to take positive action. Any action taken is often a 'knee jerk' response without assessment, to fulfil a political agenda in order to appear to be taking action in a major crisis. So often this leads to failure and disillusionment.

Fortunately there are ways in which pressures can be identified and needs assessed, to provide an appropriate support system. Figure 2.2 summarises some of the short term effects on an individual of an imbalance between pressures or demands and responses. It also shows how the cumulative effect can have longer term implications as it spreads to the family, home, social life and the workplace and wider community.

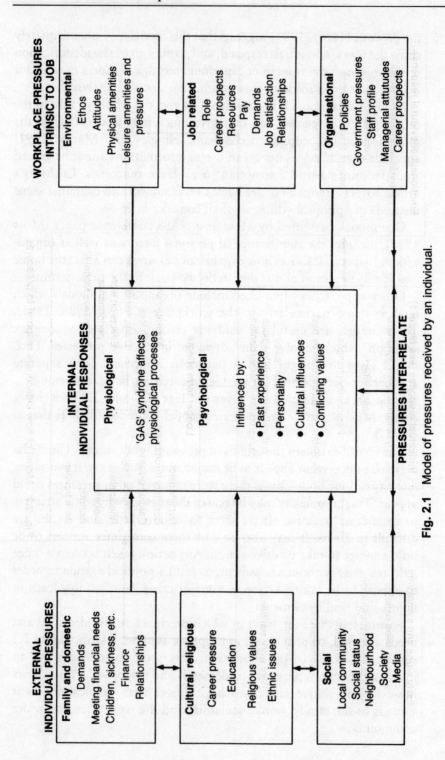

Fig. 2.1 Model of pressures received by an individual.

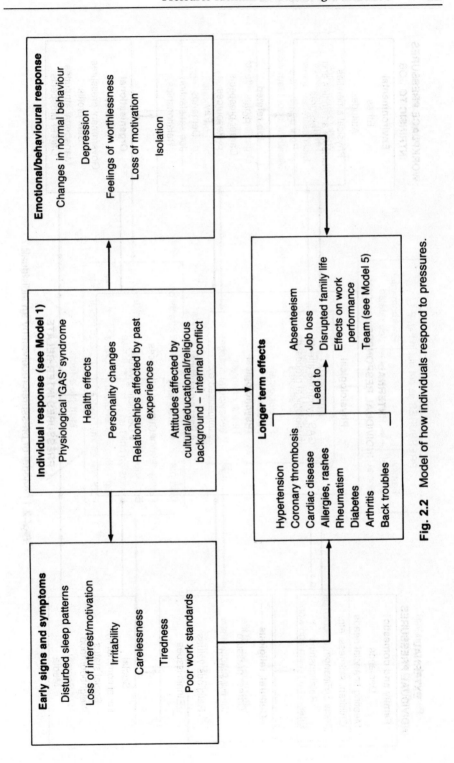

Fig. 2.2 Model of how individuals respond to pressures.

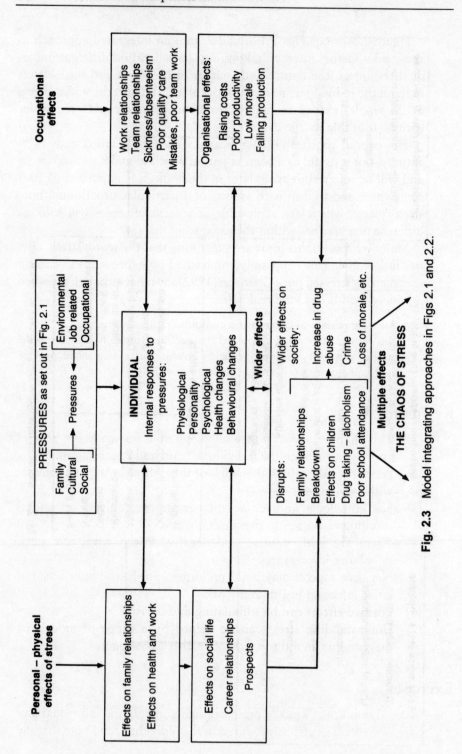

Occupational effects

Work relationships
Team relationships
Sickness/absenteeism
Poor quality care
Mistakes, poor team work

Organisational effects:
Rising costs
Poor productivity
Low morale
Falling production

PRESSURES as set out in Fig. 2.1

Environmental
Job related
Occupational

Family
Cultural
Social

Pressures

INDIVIDUAL

Internal responses to pressures:

Physiological
Personality
Psychological
Health changes
Behavioural changes

Wider effects

Wider effects on society:

Increase in drug abuse
Crime
Loss of morale, etc.

Disrupts:

Family relationships
Breakdown
Effects on children
Drug taking – alcoholism
Poor school attendance

Multiple effects
THE CHAOS OF STRESS

Personal – physical effects of stress

Effects on family relationships
Effects on health and work

Effects on social life
Career relationships
Prospects

Fig. 2.3   Model integrating approaches in Figs 2.1 and 2.2.

Figure 2.3 brings Figs 2.1. and 2.2. into an integrated approach to show how factors interact, taking into consideration different individual responses, the nature and sources of pressures and their effects both on the individual and in the workplace, and also the wider effects as the ripples extend to family, team, organisation and even wider society, resulting in 'the chaos of stress'.

This overall approach is complicated if used for detailed study in its entirety, but is useful as a context within which to make an assessment and will be referred to again later in the book. It is important to start somewhere and to deal with aspects of a particular situation in 'bite-sized' pieces which are achievable. The next chapters will look at different *perspectives* within the same scenario.

Many writers on this topic are suggesting that the word 'stress' now has little value. This is possibly emphasised by expressions in current use, such as 'stressed out'. Charlton (1992) says that although the word is widely used it has little real value:

'... serving mainly to confuse and confound rational thought...
... we should stop using the word "stress" and instead discuss specific stimuli or responses as appropriate... Pressure or tension might provide suitable substitutes for everyday clinical practice.'

Key points

(1) The chapter opens with a three point framework for general approach, through the individual, team and organisation.

(2) Pressures can arise within each of these three areas, and interact with each other.

(3) Self knowledge and self acceptance are prerequisites for understanding responses to pressures.

(4) There are both positive and negative effects from too much imbalance in pressures.

(5) Negative aspects may build up imperceptibly and have a cumulative effect on health and work.

(6) Positive effects can be stimulating and creative.

(7) Understanding stress can be helped by a range of models or diagrams as an aid to study or further assessment.

Exercises

(2.1) Look at the kind of pressures that confront the individual and the kind of effects produced in the individual, and note that the pressures are not entirely in the occupational setting. Then consider how those pressures can affect the individual, remembering that individuals respond in different ways.

(2.2)   List some of your own responses to stressful situations, both positive and negative. Put them aside for reference later on.

(2.3)   List some of your personal strengths which could prove valuable in combating the effects of stress.

(2.4)   Quote a situation from your own experience when you have noticed two people responding differently to a traumatic situation.

You may like to use exercises 2.1 and 2.4 as points for a group discussion, making notes on your observations.

Chapter 3

Practicalities and Perspectives – Minimising the Impact

The first step towards minimising the impact of stress is to accept it as an *integral feature* of normal life. Taking practical steps to deal with it, however, can be more complex than envisaged, involving:

- Acknowledgement that there are stressful situations which can have harmful effects
- Identification of specific pressures and the nature of their impact
- Identification of the causes and origins of the stressors for individuals, teams and the organisation as a whole
- Identification of personal sources of stress for individuals.

For any manager analysing overall levels of stress in staff generally and in individuals in particular, it will be possible to move on to identify with each member of staff the sources of their own stressors. This early identification should enable the individual to be involved in taking responsibility for handling their personal stressors and to play a creative role in addressing team or organisational stressors.

Some stressors arise from the individual's internal responses or home and family pressures, while others are inherent in the job and working environment. Some are communal and arise from the wider working organisation, while others relate to factors outside the work situation. It is important to analyse these stressors and their contribution to the overall levels of stress, to look carefully at them in a more complex way than is often envisaged, and to categorise them broadly before embarking on support provisions. There are stressors which affect everyone in that particular environment or profession, and those that are variable and particular to each individual.

A framework for assessment of stress levels

A framework of assessment can be applied in several different ways but it is difficult to convey this in a two-dimensional diagram. For example, the starting point for the assessor will vary according to the assessor's position in the hierarchical structure (see Fig. 3.4.).

When looking at stress and stressful situations, individuals begin with a *personal view* applicable to that particular time. An individual often blames their job for any pressure, and therefore a managerial or therapeutic assessment made from a different starting point will present a different perspective. Full assessment involves taking into consideration the nature of the job, its demands and pressures, team roles, responsibilities and working relationships, as well as the individual's interpretation of the role and their personal capacity to fulfil that role.

The whole scenario can be assessed in two main sections:

(1)   Assessing the total work situation
(2)   Assessing the particular job.

Analysing the total situation

A framework of assessment for a particular situation will need several different starting points, as stressors arise from different origins. The principle in this book has been to start with the individual person. Here the assessment will consider:

• The individual involved
• The team involved and the relationships within that team
• The organisational management.

A basic framework for assessment of pressures and needs is introduced here to act as a point of reference (Fig. 3.1) and will be developed to explore all aspects involved. It will later serve as a framework for identifying needs and deciding on priorities (Chapter 6).

The steps in analysis of the situation are:

• To identify those stressors which can be lessened by the *individual* because they are created by that person's own lifestyle, understanding and attitudes
• To look at those stressors which can be removed by improving the method of *management* or by some *adaptation* in the working environment
• To identify those which can be lessened by *adaptation of the individual* or by improved *management within the team*

- To find out those pressures which are inherent in the situation and *unavoidable* and therefore need specific support provision.

Within this process three areas of prevention are now recognised (Cooper *et al.* 1996) as:

(1) *Primary prevention* – taking action to reduce or eliminate stressors
(2) *Secondary prevention* – increasing stress awareness and assisting employees to manage stress effectively
(3) *Tertiary prevention* – provision for individuals who have suffered from serious effects of stress.

Where reduction of stressors is not possible this should not be regarded with despair, but shows the need for greater levels of commitment and creative thinking on the part of management, the team and each individual. This co-operative approach enables the best systems for coping to be identified and implemented in the team and by the individual, thus preventing the impairment of function associated with stress.

This is an ongoing management process, both in terms of management of personal response and general management of work, and involves principles which can be applied to personal life as well. Within all of this there is a wide range of knowledge, skills and resources which can be used in response to need. The process of selecting the most efficient resources is far from straightforward. This is apparent from looking at lists of pressures, which are often presented with the assumption that they are common to all situations. Clearly a wide range of general, built-in services is essential, but their use can be much more cost effective and helpful to the recipient if a careful assessment of need is available. The same pressures may be perceived differently by different individuals or groups, and as we shall see later the intensity of their effects may well be very different also.

A *practical assessment tool*

With a *managerial approach* there is assessment of the *job* and of *the team*, both in the sense of where they are now and whether they are likely to change in the future. This takes us back to the categories mentioned earlier of pressures which can be eradicated or minimised and those which cannot be altered. It is necessary to 'juggle' with an overlapping set of assessment factors, such as *selection* – assessment of the person's suitability – *training and development* facilities, *educational needs*, and *support mechanisms* to equip the person to do the job. Another factor is the quality of the *culture of care* which needs to cascade through all levels of the organisation and should be taken into account in any assessment. A common understanding is necessary of the criteria used for this assessment, and a policy of response to the assessment of pressures is needed. If support mechanisms are identified throughout the organisation this helps to educate staff, encouraging the establishment of caring attitudes in all departments. If criteria are established and articulated, awareness and recognition will be increased, both of need and response. This will improve communication and make it effective, understood and manageable.

A major difficulty is that language is understood differently by different professions and groups of staff.

'For the failure of language
there is no redress. The physicists
tell us your size, the chemists the ingredients of your
thinking. But who you are
does not appear, nor why
on the innocent marches
of vocabulary, you should choose
to engage us, belabouring us with your silence.'

R.S. Thomas: *The Combat*

An assessment may be proactive, such as to make an informed approach to planning and creating a healthy workplace, or it may be reactive, made in the light of problems which have arisen. For example, a member of staff may be showing signs of excessive stress as a response to pressure, or there may be an increase in stress related illness or absenteeism.

It may be useful to assess the levels of stressful responses of staff in particular units or vulnerable areas, for which a 'stress inventory' or 'stress check' list may be used. A number of these are available, such as the MSF Stress Kit (MSF 1995), or others listed in various texts such as Cartwright & Cooper (1994). These may not produce scientifically accurate results because of variables which are difficult to control. For example, if the checks are made at different times, different moods may influence results and present a false sense of gloom or euphoria; or a change of staff or threat of change of roles may create a higher level of stress than normal.

Identifying and managing stress

The first stage of any analysis of stress must be to identify its origins in that particular workplace. In setting up a framework for this we use our three distinct perspectives from which an analysis should be made:

(1) from the individual's perspective
(2) from the team's perspective
(3) from the managerial perspective.

Figure 3.1 shows the overall framework for analysis. The process of assessment will involve looking at the specific areas shown in Figs 3.2 and 3.3. Finally the particular assessments will need to be considered in

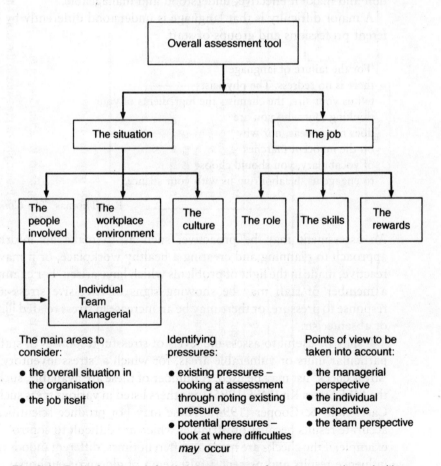

Fig. 3.1 Basic framework for the assessment of pressures and needs (the contents of each box are further broken down into detail later in the text and in Figs 3.2 and 3.3).

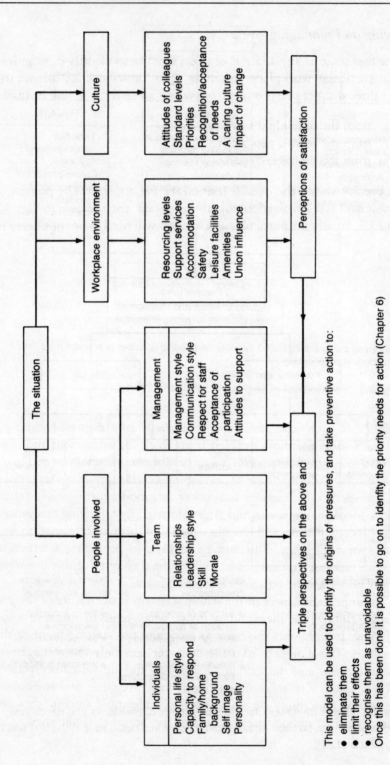

Fig. 3.2 Assessment of the origins of pressure in the work situation.

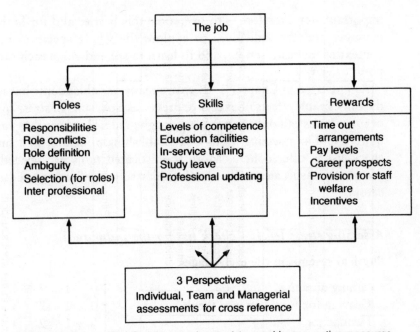

Fig. 3.3   Assessment of origins of pressure in the job.

relation to each other, to identify the origins of pressures. Figures 3.2 and 3.3 show the more detailed framework for assessment and *identification of stressors* and their source in the *work situation* and in the *specific job*. As the process of developing a staff support system unfolds (Chapters 5 to 8), various sections of this model form a basic framework for *assessing needs*, and later priorities. By following this process a composite picture will emerge which will form an information base for a strategic plan. This will be realistic in providing a structural service tailored to local needs, and the final chapter of this book will show how these fit into an integrated pattern.

An important aspect of the whole scenario is the nature of the *prevailing culture*, the 'them and us' divide which tends to influence points of view. It highlights the need to recognise the starting point in this analysis. The danger is that the manager sees only the management point of view and the individual sees only the individual perspective. Where the ability to communicate is lost, prejudice and resentment grow and the ability or willingness to understand one another and discover a common ground is lost or severely diminished. One important step therefore is to overcome this barrier and for both the manager and the individual to explore the whole spectrum in the context of the team setting, and to learn to see and value each other's point of view.

As indicated in Chapter 2, there are many variables contributing to the undesirable effects of excessive pressures, so results of *stress checks* or *inventories* can only be used as a rough guide. However they can be quite useful in assessing needs and establishing priorities, so a simple check list is offered here. More sophisticated tools are needed for accurate measurement. This list includes some well recognised indicators.

Assessing stress levels – check list for the individual

Physical systems in the early stages

Failing appetite	0	1	2	3	4
Craving for food between meals	0	1	2	3	4
Headaches	0	1	2	3	4
Muscle cramps	0	1	2	3	4
Indigestion	0	1	2	3	4
Sweating of palms at night	0	1	2	3	4
Insomnia	0	1	2	3	4
Breathlessness	0	1	2	3	4
Raised blood pressure	0	1	2	3	4
Skin rashes	0	1	2	3	4

Emotional or psychological symptoms

Irritability	0	1	2	3	4
Constant tiredness – even after sleep	0	1	2	3	4
Difficulty in decision making	0	1	2	3	4
Anxiety and tension	0	1	2	3	4
Panics	0	1	2	3	4
Feelings of failure	0	1	2	3	4
Feeling 'unable to cope'	0	1	2	3	4
Concentration difficulties	0	1	2	3	4
Loss of interest in life	0	1	2	3	4
Feeling bored or depressed	0	1	2	3	4

Behavioural/social symptoms

Increased alcohol consumption or smoking	0	1	2	3	4
Increasing depression	0	1	2	3	4

Difficult relationships at work	0	1	2	3	4
Becoming withdrawn	0	1	2	3	4
Unable to face criticism	0	1	2	3	4
Carelessness in dress and appearance	0	1	2	3	4
Increased tendency for accidents	0	1	2	3	4

These are some of the early signs of the cumulative effects of excessive pressures. It is not only the total score that is important, but areas with high scores, such as 3 or 4, which are those needing most attention. It is also useful when cross referencing results from different people (provided the same check list is used), to note the scores which are high from all individuals and therefore indicate areas needing urgent attention.

Stress at work
A similar check list can be used to identify a particular source of stress in the workplace. It can help to identify areas of concern, especially if different perspectives are taken into account.

Origins of pressure

Long working hours	0	1	2	3	4
Working unpopular shifts	0	1	2	3	4
Job insecurity	0	1	2	3	4
Inadequate professional updating	0	1	2	3	4
Role conflicts	0	1	2	3	4
Conflicts of loyalty	0	1	2	3	4
Conflict between personal values and practices required	0	1	2	3	4
Responsibility – too little, too much	0	1	2	3	4
Lack of career prospects	0	1	2	3	4
Financial worries – inadequate pay	0	1	2	3	4
Information overload	0	1	2	3	4
Dealing with death, disability etc.	0	1	2	3	4
Dealing with distressed relatives	0	1	2	3	4
Lack of support or supervision	0	1	2	3	4
Risks of physical violence	0	1	2	3	4
Work relationships – difficulty with colleagues	0	1	2	3	4
Management styles	0	1	2	3	4
Communication channels	0	1	2	3	4
Feeling undervalued	0	1	2	3	4

Patient and public expectations	0	1	2	3	4
Fears of litigation	0	1	2	3	4
Boredom	0	1	2	3	4
Poor working conditions	0	1	2	3	4
Too many meetings	0	1	2	3	4
Too many deadlines	0	1	2	3	4

From the individual's perspective

Individual personality

Each individual has a unique set of experiences, beliefs and environmental influences in the early years of life, which contribute to the formation of a unique personality. Early learning experiences and relationships are also a vital element in the process of shaping attitudes and the kind of person we become. About 50% of intellectual growth occurs during a most sensitive period of development up to four years old (Kellner-Pringle 1975). There are several different approaches to the importance of early bonding processes; these may seem contradictory but help our understanding of the concept of personality formation as it contributes to our resilience and response to pressures in later life.

- The *psychological approach* concentrates on the importance of bonding effectively in the early years (Foss 1961, 1963; Rutter 1972; Storr 1981).
- *Learning theories* look at the importance of stimulus and response in the development of behaviour patterns (Elkin 1960; Rogers 1967). There is a Swedish study which has demonstrated that nurses who were well loved and had satisfactory relationships in their early years were much better able to respond positively to stressful situations at work.
- There is also the *sociological perspective* which looks at primary and secondary socialisation in relation to influences from families and groups and cultural influences in personality formation (White 1977).
- There is also an important effect due to *previous life experiences* such as loss, death or trauma of any kind, which if not resolved at the time of the event can have a long term effect on the individual's response to particular situations.

These approaches are all illuminating when studying the different responses to pressure attributable to personality differences.

The individual tends to consider the self first, set in the context of the family and social setting, then the job and aspects of job satisfaction, and after that the team and the working environment. Thus many elements may be related for the individual, and just as managers will start from their own perspective to assess the pressures, so the individual starting from a different perspective will look at similar issues in quite a different light in terms of the personal pressures likely to be experienced. While the manager analyses what happens to the job, the individual's priority is, 'What will it do to me?'; 'What will it do to my patients?'. For the individual the perspective starts with self and job satisfaction and the effect on his own life, socially, at home and professionally; whereas the manager says, 'What effect does this have on the service?'.

In ideal circumstances the individual wants a satisfying job that fulfils personal needs and values, fully uses personal skills, and gives a sense of self worth; while the manager asks what it contributes towards the task being accomplished and will the desired outcomes be achieved? This could be an area of potential conflict as the manager looks, for example, for the highest throughput of patients at the lowest possible cost, while the individual wants personal and professional job satisfaction.

The job itself as part of the team

The individual has expectations from the job, asking for instance whether it will enable the bills to be paid, whether it will enable social life to be maintained. A priority will be delivering the highest standard of care to patients and relatives. Constant irritations can result from staff reductions which lead to curtailment of some aspects of care.

The individual may also be assessing how fellow professionals, colleagues and carers work together to achieve their aims and may look to them to provide support, understanding and encouragement, and to share the same broad priorities. The working environment will be viewed as the place which enables work to be carried out and patient care to be given. A negative aspect arises when jobs are under threat and competition with colleagues may result, creating defensive attitudes which lead to poor relationships and diminish team performance and satisfaction.

The working environment needs to be user friendly, for the team as well as the patients and relatives; it also needs to be functional and supportive of the team's needs. In the absence of a suitable environment there is stress and alienation from the job and management, and a feeling of being undervalued.

From the managerial perspective

Perspective on the job (Fig. 3.3)

The job itself is often blamed by the occupant for any stress, therefore an objective managerial or therapeutic assessment needs to be made of all aspects of it.

Looking at the job means evaluating carefully the job to be done. This has to be set in the context of the team and department, which in turn has to be set in the context of the whole organisation. As aims and objectives are set out for the team and department, each job can be evaluated and described effectively.

From the managerial perspective this will include the nature of the job, its demands and pressures, the level of responsibility, relationships with other workers, the interests of the department, and the individual's own interpretation of the role and their personal capacity to fill that role. It will include such general factors as:

- The level of teamwork required, including how exacting the job is in terms of relationships
- The qualifications and skill levels required
- The need to take responsibility for others
- The potential pressures, both mentally and physically.

Other useful factors relate to the special nature of the job, such as:

- Isolation, geographical or professional, which may indicate the level of team support to be expected
- The nature of the work in terms of stimulation or boredom – e.g. is it repetitive?
- Does it require initiative and innovation?
- Does it involve travelling or frequent contact with other agencies?

These are just a few of the factors to take into account to get the match right between the person and the job, and also to assess the vulnerable areas where pressures are likely to arise and to build in appropriate preventive measures and support.

The working environment

The working environment plays an important part in the cultural organisation. *Managerially* the overall ethos of the organisation is primarily dictated by the prevailing government and health department policies and directives. This includes the setting of targets, policies and budgets, which reflect the government viewpoint on priorities in health care, and the relative importance of the needs of different groups of patients and families. Specific directives set standards to be reached, and these must be translated into action at trust level. Staff views, as transmitted through teams and professional groups, are also incorporated, and other influences include working conditions and pay policies.

The local working environment and organisational culture is affected by the national culture and by local interpretation of national guidelines. The complex nature of purchasers' interpretation of national guidlelines, taking into account fundholding GPs and the fact that decisions over funding are often communicated at a late stage, makes management of the provision of services difficult. It can also be affected by whether the trust is dealing with one area or is a complex trust with subregional specialities relating to several district purchasers; and by the nature of the community serviced by the trust, e.g. whether it is a deprived area or one with many multicultural needs.

The internal aspect of the individual trust, which includes inter-relationships between different departments, and the relative levels of resourcing and priorities in allocation of resources, can cause severe problems in relationships. Figure 3.4 shows that assessments can go in two directions: from the top down (e.g. from the manager) or from the bottom up (e.g. from the individual at any level of responsibility).

Looking at the team

Each team is set within the context of the organisation, the working environment and the particular task, and is affected by the quality of relationships within the team. So this part of the assessment will be different for different departments and can even vary between two departments of similar nature. The level of stress generated within any team, and the way it is managed, can have a considerable effect on the creativity and productivity of that team, and the wellbeing of

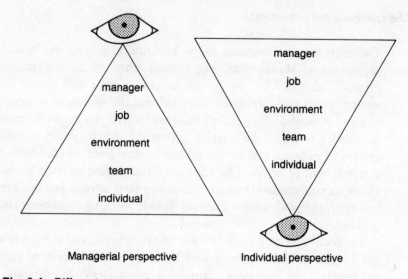

Fig. 3.4 Different perspectives on staff support.

individuals making up the team. The manager needs to create a team within which individual members' skills are enhanced by the interactions within the team. This ensures that the highest quality of care and productivity is maintained, and the essential elements of the function are carried out effectively. The team environment needs to be created so that ideas can be generated, evaluated, allocated and put into practice.

Team relationships are vital. Negative relationships create fear and anxiety and have a downward spiral effect (Stoter 1991) which results in a lowering of achievement, poor job satisfaction and resentment. This may lead to the development of separate factions within the team, as individuals feel isolated and start acting independently and sniping at the management and each other, creating a tense and unpleasant working environment.

In a team with good relationships stress is minimised and there is cohesion. Good relationships increase motivation and team loyalties, creating a pleasant working environment which enhances job satisfaction and reduces absenteeism and sickness rates.

Identifying stress origins means identifying the factors which create a lack of cohesion, and the pressures which jar and grate and lead to secrecy, often indicating a seeking of power and control as information is guarded and kept from the team, leading to resentment and the breakdown of communication.

Looking at the individual

When considering the individual, the manager needs to acknowledge the many factors which influence the level of stress and the ability to respond to it: personality, culture, home and family background and circumstances, the work situation, and the social arena. All these factors affect the individual with a range of demands and pressures and interact with each other to affect the stress levels. It is important to understand each individual's capacity to respond in a positive or negative manner to pressures. This response can be enhanced or negated to a considerable extent by the culture of the organisation, by the relationships within the team and by the support available. These factors should be assessed to enable managers to communicate effectively and appropriately and to provide the best support systems for each situation.

This overall perspective from the manager's point of view covers a wide range of factors, and the alternative approach then needs to be taken to look at the same issues from the individual's perspective.

Looking at the job

The job itself is viewed by the manager in relation to other parts of the organisation, but is seen differently by the individual. Pressures are created when the needs of other parts of the organisation seem to be rated more highly and appear in conflict. Perceptions differ between individuals with different roles or levels of responsibility. The ward sister has different views from the student or the unit manager, especially where units are suffering from competition for scarce resources. In this situation staff at the lower levels can feel undervalued as they feel the patient suffers and their contribution to service is undervalued.

Stress generated in these circumstances is cumulative and permeates all aspects of the job and the teams. The manager will hopefully weigh up all aspects and respond appropriately. When this is done well it is possible to eliminate some stressors, to minimise others, or to provide built-in support where the stressors are inherent in the job. An essential ingredient in this process of minimising the effect of pressure and stress must be to maintain dialogue between all concerned at all times. This is a major aspect of support, as discussed later.

Perspectives of managers and individuals when assessed together will merge and be reflected in the team performance, which is one ultimate goal. A good, healthy team has the ability to help with integrating the management and individual perspectives. The team is the first drawing together of individuals within a specific area or place of work, and has the duty to respond to the policies created at management level and translate them into action to provide an effective service. It draws individuals from being just individuals into co-operating with others to create an effective response to the needs of patients, and to implement the policies of management and cope with the limitation of resources.

Integration of different perspectives

Following on from the specific way of looking at situations, as individuals and management, an integrated response is needed to avoid the development of resentment and the attitude of 'them and us' which exists so often between management and individuals. An integrated model of approach can weigh up and bring together the needs of the organisation and the individuals, and recognise the inter-relationship of the pressures affecting each.

To create a healthy environment in the workplace, all these perspectives need to be seen and understood by every individual involved, with respect for each other's perspectives. This integration is about finding the means of valuing individuals and teams (rather than 'making them feel valued' – there is a difference) so that patient care follows naturally from having created a caring and healthy working environment which values and respects people.

This is what integration and good patient care is about. One of the key factors is to get the right people into the right jobs, as each individual has an effect on the team and through the team on the whole organisation. An unsuitable appointment can have a profound impact on the ability of the team to give a good service. Clearly this issue becomes more important in more senior posts, but even at junior levels an unsuitable appointment can create a lack of trust which is damaging to effective team work. It is thus crucial to recognise the work the team does and the role of each individual performance within the team, and to ensure that an accurate job specification is drawn up with a clear person specification, to ensure the right person is appointed.

This demands a clear recognition of the role of the team and the way the team functions. Recognition also needs to be given to differences in ostensibly similar teams, as the teams may be very different due to the different individuals which make up each team. Careful selection needs to be applied to ensure the right appointment is made, then that person needs to be given proper support to develop the skills and abilities to do the job, and to be integrated into the team and organisation. Therefore a good orientation programme needs to be planned, relating to the ethos of the team and the way the team relates to the rest of the organisation. A well thought out, continuing education programme is an important part of team building and staff support.

Other points of view (source unknown)

'I was standing once in an airport ticket line behind two children, brother and sister, neither one over 9 years old. They were fighting over an ice cream cone. The flavour was a gooey concoction called "bubble gum" with real chunks of gum buried in the ice cream. In front of them oblivious of their struggle was a woman in a mink coat. This was an accident waiting to happen. I considered stepping in telling the kids to be careful, that they might smear ice cream over the coat. Then I heard the girl tell the boy, "If you don't stop Charlie, you'll have hairs from that lady's coat on your cone!"'

Key points

(1) The damaging effects of stress may be limited or eliminated once the sources are identified

(2) A framework for assessment is a useful tool to aid identification of pressure points

(3) There are different perspectives from which to view these issues – managerial and individual

(4) It is vital to consider these two perspectives together when identifying the origins of potentially stressful situations

(5) Selection of the right person for a post is vital.

Exercises

(3.1) Consider your own sphere of work and identify some of the origins of pressure which could be eliminated, limited or require support to minimise.

(3.2) By what means could these pressures have been avoided? You may find this topic suitable for a group discussion or as part of your personal development record.

Chapter 4

Different Perspectives on Practical Pressures

The nature and origins of the pressures generating undesirable levels of stress have been explored in previous chapters from the point of view of individuals, managers and teams. These have related to pressures in the structural setting but there are other dimensions that need to be considered if an accurate identification of pressures is to be made, and appropriate preventive and supportive measures are to be taken. Sometimes support services are set up and later abandoned. This is because the mechanisms offered are unrelated to the situation concerned and do not meet specific needs, and so the results fail to meet the employer's expectations. The horticultural example below may offer an interesting illustration.

Any garden-lover planning a new garden from scratch will do well to discover any *special features* about local conditions. Analysis of the soil and a knowledge of weather conditions, prevailing winds or average rainfall will guide the planner on the kind of plants to use and the sort of soil treatment which will encourage good growth. Such careful planning will save much waste of time and resources and avoid many failures and disappointments. The analysis, preparation and care in choice facilitates the growth, integration and success of the plants.

Similarly, proper assessment of specific pressures for a particular group will help prevent many of the damaging effects of stress and create a good working environment as a basis for a healthy workforce. Interest is increasing in identifying the origins of stress in different occupations as the health of the workforce is becoming a matter for concern. A comparison between different occupations and work settings shows that while some pressures are common to all, most have particular features related to the nature of the job. Health care occupations are clearly stressful by nature as staff are constantly dealing with life and death crises, suffering and bereavement – matters that are distressing to all humans.

The field of health care is a popular one for research studies related to stress, especially in professions like nursing where it is not difficult to obtain a good sized sample and where a range of specialities offers scope for comparison. Areas attracting attention include, for example, intensive care and accident and emergency, paediatric and neonatal care, and psychiatric, community nursing and hospice care, while areas such as geriatric care or rehabilitation receive scant attention. Education in medical and nursing professions is frequently studied, and specialist areas such as HIV are becoming popular for observations of staff pressures.

Most studies tend to identify the usual pressures, common to health care, such as:

- Concern over lack of resources, leading to inability to maintain standards
- Poor working environment
- Traumatic incidents
- Feelings of being undervalued.

Different specialities do throw up some *particular pressures* although many do not show significant differences. For example:

- A study by Carlisle *et al.* (1994) found that midwives suffered from role ambiguity, particularly when that role was confused with nursing, and they experienced a loss of autonomy
- Hinds *et al.* (1994) noticed that the more experienced nurses in paediatrics reported fewer pressures from their work
- Scullion (1994) in A&E departments recorded that the age of the nurse was not relevant to the degree of stress
- In groups like those working with HIV sufferers, researchers found conflict was generated by problems relating to confidentiality (Miller 1995)
- Death and bereavement appeared to be cited as pressures in most studies, particularly where children were concerned (Scullion 1994; Downey *et al.* 1995)
- Menon's study on managers (Menon & Akhilesh 1994) reinforced an observation made earlier that many pressures could be eliminated or at least controlled if they were identified

- Aurelio (1993) observed the other side of the coin: that an optimum level of pressure leads to high job satisfaction as it sets off those very coping mechanisms which can be stressors.

In medicine the groups commonly studied are GPs, who find that the changes in community practices cause confusion, or junior doctors who work a notoriously high number of hours.

These examples are selected from a range of well conducted studies which make a useful contribution to this field of study but do not show the whole picture. Any reader wishing to explore a particular occupation should consult the original papers for a full account. It is important to recognise that as they are isolated subjects, general assumptions cannot be made from them and they must be assessed in the context for which they were intended. This reinforces the necessity for assessment in *local* situations, as described in the previous chapter. It is also a good reason for making an assessment in the light of experience in the real life setting, taking into account the prevailing culture of the day and the working environment. We will now explore some situations with which many of us are familiar.

New entrants to the caring services

The majority of people entering the caring services do so as students of a particular profession, and therefore are most likely to be young and starting out on their careers. There is, however, an increasing trend for more mature people to enter the professions. They may be vulnerable to the same professional pressures, but they are facing these from a quite different standpoint as they bring an accumulation of experience from their own particular life experience.

Young students

Young students enter a profession having decided what they want to do with their lives, which is likely to include 'doing something for other people'. They come from an educational environment where they have been used to considerable freedom, especially at the more senior level, and this particularly applies to university entrants. They have been encouraged to choose what they do – to select the essay subjects and when to do the work, and to decide which lectures to attend as not all are compulsory. But at work they are entering a situation which makes considerable demands and where the flexibility and opportunity to make choices is more limited, as they move into an environment where actions and decisions are influenced by other people's demands and preferences, particularly those of patients and relatives. They are confronted by new and different sets of values and trust, which make a deep impact, together with new responsibilities at a stage of personal development when beliefs, understanding and personal relationships may be volatile. It may well be difficult to take proper care of themselves and achieve a balance between past and present values, and to integrate work and social activity without support.

The *interaction* between important aspects of development can lead to powerful emotions and tensions and can have an impact on health in terms of eating and sleeping habits, and undermining confidence and a sense of security. There is also an existing environment which often presents a 'them and us' culture between individuals and senior staff.

Feelings of isolation may occur as higher levels of responsibility are given with little support and back-up, creating new pressures. Part of the problem lies in the difficulty of asking for support and guidance – wondering if they will be seen to be failures for not coping – and recognising that those they turn to for support appear too busy. It takes courage to ask questions, and a sense of maturity and confidence to admit that they 'don't know'.

There is often the added *unsettling situation* where students are moved between different sites and units to acquire different experiences, so becoming separated from familiar friends and places. This constant movement creates a feeling of 'not belonging' anywhere, and living in an atmosphere of constant change in a scene of new relationships and environments often leads to a sense of insecurity. The student may experience an undermining of self-worth through lack of knowledge as they enter new situations.

There are also pressures to *achieve results*, both in the academic and practical sense, and to reach professional standards while facing constant peer group pressures. Antipathy may exist between different student groups as their paths cross and diverge. There can be areas of non-acceptance and even rivalry between groups, and often the prevailing culture 'them and us' attitudes is reflected between groups.

There are many pressures common to all young people within domestic and social relationships as they seek to survive on basic living standards and low incomes. Many have had a protective home life where everything was provided, and they have to adjust to budgeting and planning carefully how to manage for themselves, all in the context of a working life with a disciplined schedule. They face a life in a large institutional setting planned around other people's lives and needs.- They move from a relatively sheltered existence into a place where everything focuses on a section of the population which is faced with big challenges of life and death, and they meet lives devastated through disease, accident, disfiguration and death.

Mature students

For the mature student many of these pressures are encountered for the first time at an older age as they enter a scene of challenge and change, facing new values. All this is in the context of past experience and ideals, and mixed with the fear of 'not making it' or doubts about their ability to cope, with the threat of possible job loss at the end, or insecurity about their ability to change direction and apply existing knowledge to their professional skills. However, they can bring reserves from past experience which can be an asset in helping them to make adjustments. Personal responsibilities may be at a different level, with growing families who make demands on their time and attention. They meet their pressures from a somewhat different perspective, while at the same time having to adjust to the authority of younger staff who are more highly skilled professionally.

Specific professional pressures

Pressures tend to change, diminish or increase with greater seniority in the organisation. In a large institution with a medical and nursing and other schools attached, there is a constant flow of students at various stages of their professional education. During the earlier years there are the common pressures associated with studying and taking exams, and balancing this with new relationships and establishing an active social life. As time passes there are greater challenges as staff are confronted with suffering, and with possible challenges to their ideals and beliefs in the face of suffering. There are pressures of learning to take responsibility, ethical pressures and pressures of decision making where there may be conflict within themselves as well as with other professionals. Some of these issues are common to all groups as they move towards more responsibility. Mature students will face them with different backgrounds of experience and will therefore respond differently.

There are, however, some pressures which are specific to particular professions. For example, there is the problem much publicised in the press of long hours of duty for young doctors during their years in junior posts. There are important decisions to be made concerning careers, whether to pursue a medical or surgical path or move into the community or the mental health fields. Nurses and others may well have to face similar dilemmas as they decide on future careers. There is constant rivalry among students following more academic or specialist courses, where false assumptions may be made. For example, student nurses following degree courses find themselves considered incompetent practitioners by colleagues of all professions, when in fact there is strong evidence to the contrary (Owen 1988). Many degree students in the caring professions are considered to be elitist groups who will never make 'good practitioners', and therefore they often lack confidence or may give other colleagues a feeling of inferiority. Such attitudes serve to perpetuate the 'them and us' culture met so often and built on false attitudes and assumptions.

Professionals, as they progress along career paths, are expected to take on more and more responsibility for themselves, patients, families and other members of staff. The number of complexities to be juggled at any one time increases.

As a student most will have had one or a few patients only to deal with at any one time, whereas the ward or team leader has a more extended role, dealing with other people within a team of professionals and maintaining overall responsibility of care. There are pressures related to financial contracts and ethical and technological aspects, balancing care between the demands in the ward, not only for the individual but for the professional team. At the same time there are pressures to remain effective in practice.

There is more teaching responsibility with its ethical problems and the need to stay in the forefront of knowledge. There is the responsibility of passing on this knowledge effectively, and the need to find time to keep up to date with reading. Teachers and clinicians may find it difficult to combine teaching and practice skills as they attempt to combine the skills and attitudes of two different worlds. Those purely in practice must balance the knowledge of what is desirable with what is possible, and must focus on what is available. This may limit their performance and create many inner tensions and frustrations, particularly for those with a wider vision and a desire to give a first class service.

Moving between different areas and fields of work, which function differently, brings its own pressures, with new parameters and the need to adapt practice. There are many pressures of adaptability and social upheaval between colleagues, friends, different housing, etc. Support mechanisms are disrupted and new ones need to be established, together with new relationships.

Doctors have particular responsibility, and therefore pressures, in decision making, diagnosis and prescribing treatment in difficult cases.

Managers

Managers have the overall responsibility of managing the organisation or unit. In senior management all areas of expertise have to be balanced against the overall aims of the organisation. There are pressures to deliver what is laid down by government and the health department within rapidly changing targets and against a political background where targets can be moved, especially in a period where a general election is anticipated.

Managers must negotiate with financial committees and district health commissions, who set priorities and allocate resources. This creates uncertainty and difficulties for long term planning as restrictions or regular demands for savings are imposed. Managers are under pressure – if they do not deliver, they lose their jobs; and there is the responsibility for many other jobs if targets are not met, with redundancies a reality. The overall responsibility for effective delivery of care in the statutory services increases the area of pressure for both managers and professionals, as they look at and plan the service.

Community staff

Community staff experience pressures peculiar to the nature of their work environment or their professional practice. Some pressures are due to isolation, caused by a remote location or by working in a small team where they are isolated from other professionals of their own disciplines. There are pressures arising from the need to liaise with other professions, voluntary groups and local government staff and administrators. Community staff may also find pressures arising from being unable to offer the quality of care they are committed to with families or patients, where resources are limited. They often find themselves on the receiving end of anger, rage or even violence, which can be very stressful. They may often feel that their special needs are not being met.

Ancillary workers

Ancillary workers cover administrative, clerical and maintenance staff.

- Administrative staff are under pressure from managers as there is a conflict between tight internal controls and the levels of staffing required to do the work
- They are also in competition with professionals
- The number of reports required by government and administrative systems is very high when administrative costs need to be reduced
- There is a need to communicate, for the smooth running of care and treatment for patients, which needs good back-up support. It is vital for these staff to keep up their skills in information technology
- Ancillary workers may well be grappling with the pressures of low pay and its consequence for their families
- There is the need to keep the place functioning by cleaning, maintenance and repair. Equipment wears out more quickly as the level of funding is decreased
- Pressures on the individual grow as they feel their group is at the bottom of the pile and they are affected by political statements which appear to devalue the importance of support work.

Ambulance workers

Groups such as ambulance staff are especially vulnerable to the effects of traumatic incidents and therefore are often more exposed to the attentions of the media and general public, which brings its own pressures. Stressful incidents occur frequently, together with the unpredictability of events, such as moving between the routine work of ferrying patients home and attending a major accident or emergency needing an urgent and skilled response. They also have problems of status, which sometimes occur between paramedics and professionals attending an emergency scene. They may have to face the aggression of frightened patients who tend to blame the first person on the scene for delayed arrival, when they have been delayed in heavy traffic or by misdirections.

Staff outside the National Health Service

The pressures for professionals are often considered only in the light of what we know happens in the NHS. In fact there are many staff who work in voluntary or private health care and they have similar pressures relating to their own special area of work. Such staff include a large number in hospice care, where in many ways their pressures are recognised and some provision is made by in-service training and support. Residential care is another area often forgotten, with the pressures of patients, some of whom may be unco-operative. Professional staff also work in industry, particularly in occupational health and health promotion settings, and in services such as the prison service; all these have their own specific pressures.

General principles

Throughout all these different perspectives certain basic pressures are common for all carers, including:

- Feeling undervalued
- Facing traumatic situations
- Boring or repetitive work
- Conflicting values and lack of trust
- Lack of confidence
- Poor communications
- Conflicting role situations
- Feeling overwhelmed by staff shortages
- Feeling overwhelmed by time limitations
- Isolation or geographical separation
- Difficult team relationships
- Lack of consultation
- Lack of preparation for the job
- Pressures from personal and home life.

These may vary in intensity so there has to be recognition of special needs, as well as the back-up of support services which should cover the whole organisation.

Cultural influences

We have discussed the differences between individuals in the way they respond to pressures, also the fact that a certain amount of stress is necessary to maintain optimum performance. We have focused on the more practical effects of the different kinds of pressures peculiar to health care practitioners and organisations. This must all be seen in the context of the workplace as a whole, its cultural environment and the ethos within which practice of care takes place. Attitudes of staff are very important; sometimes there is a problem of lack of understanding between different sectors of the working community, each group going its own way and fighting its own corner, with little understanding of the particular pressures affecting other individuals and groups.

A culture of distrust brings uncertainty and creates threatening situations. This can create much stress within the organisation, particularly if staff do not participate in decision making, or where communications are poor and staff feel they are not seen as a valuable resource. This creates additional pressures which often go unrecognised until a climate of hostility between staff and managers has escalated to such an extent that a climate of discontentment and conflict is evident.

Cultural influences are important and later in this book we shall be exploring the effects of the workplace culture in relation to the wider cultural context which has a profound and subtle influence on all our values. Sometimes world events change attitudes or even have a creative influence, such as war or severe deprivation. These are issues which can affect the degree of pressures and cannot be ignored completely. In other words the effect of pressures on any staff will vary, particularly as we live in a world of rapid change.

This section of the book has offered an informative approach to encourage the reader to explore other personal interests and reading on the origins and nature of pressures arising in health care. It forms a background for looking at the specific kind of staff support required to meet a range of needs, and for providing a framework for the foundation of a staff support system.

In Section III we shall see how a well-designed staff support system can be flexible enough to respond to these changing situations.

Key points

(1) There are specific pressures which vary for different groups of staff at different stages of their career.
(2) There are specific pressures for particular groups of professionals and practitioners in different settings.
(3) Some pressures are common to all health care staff, but the needs of each group must be identified in order to provide staff support which is appropriate.

Exercise

(4.1)   Have a look at any of the studies mentioned at the beginning of
this chapter, particularly those relating to your area of work or
professional skills. Do the research findings bear out your own
experience and are there any other areas you think are being
ignored?

Section III

Meeting the Pressures – Response Through Staff Support

Chapter 5

Philosophies and Policies – The Caring Culture

The nature of staff support

In Chapter 1 an example was given of the wide variety of ideas held by staff about staff support. Some were imprecise, some broad and all-embracing, while others gave a limited picture of one particular service. This indicates scope for sharpening up views if there is to be any kind of solid foundation on which to build staff support. Frequently a support service is introduced and superimposed on an organisation ill prepared to use it, on the simplistic assumption that there is a single solution. When there is little evidence of improvement the scheme is considered a waste of resources and abandoned. Such incidents show the importance of:

- Assessing needs locally
- Identifying vulnerable areas
- Identifying existing resources
- Targeting the areas of greatest need within the overall scheme.

There is a tendency to talk about *staff care* as an alternative for *staff support*. Careful scrutiny of the words 'to care' and 'to support' in the *Shorter Oxford Dictionary* discloses subtle but interesting distinctions. Definitions of to 'care' lean heavily toward ideas of 'concern', 'attention', and 'protection'. For health care staff the idea of 'nourishing' or nurturing is often used in this context. 'To support' has eleven different definitions including 'strengthening', 'providing for the maintenance of', 'furnishing sustenance for', 'giving courage or confidence to' and to 'occupy a position by the side of'. In the context of this book these differences indicate that 'support' has the more positive and proactive sense, which is more appropriate here.

The philosophy of staff support

Central to this approach is the premise that individuals need care, just as health care staff are committed to the principle that patients or clients need care. They need to recognise that they themselves are human and have a similar basic need to be cared for. Staff support is about valuing staff as a whole, as a valuable resource in the organisation, not just as single groups and teams. It is also about valuing staff as individuals who deserve respect. Staff support is about creating and developing within each individual member of staff a sense of personal worth and self respect, valuing themselves as persons. They will then be able to value their colleagues. This leads to a general sense of worth and respect within the team and organisation. Ultimately the value of patients is raised, leading to a higher quality of care for patients, family and colleagues generally. Whatever specific provision is made, whatever the service, its effectiveness depends on the clear premise of valuing individuals at all levels within the organisation.

Attention needs to be paid to wider issues than simply ensuring the right *facilities* are in place, essential though these are as an obvious demonstration of staff care, (e.g. rest rooms, leisure facilities, other staff amenities and services.) It needs to be demonstrated that the organisation's aim is to care about and for people who deliver a service, whether their role may be professional, administrative, clerical, ancillary or voluntary. *Attitudes* must be right.

Words such as *respect, valued, dignity, attitudes* and so on appear frequently in policy statements and charters, and indeed throughout this text, and for some they may seem nebulous and hollow, especially where they do not see evidence of their existence.

A meeting had been called of staff concerned with various aspects of staff support, to discuss improvements throughout the organisation, and the allocation of resources identified for this purpose. A special allocation had featured in the approved budget, which was felt to be an achievement. At the end of an enlightened discussion, the meeting was declared closed and the chairman got up to leave, when one member said, 'Excuse me but we've not dealt with a most important question. Can we make some provision for those of us here who are at the sharp end of delivering this support?'. The reply came brusquely: 'You've got the finance. You should all know how to care for yourselves. That's your problem. You shouldn't need support. I've done my bit – it's over to you'. And the chairman swept out.

A similar story came from staff in a growing trust where the chief executive officer had featured prominently in press articles as promoting excellent staff support care in the trust. Staff working in the organisation were very frustrated and lacking in motivation. They felt relationships were poor; they knew nothing about any system. While they appreciated the need for a good public image, staff at grass roots level had felt they were unimportant and no one cared about them. Even an attempt to set up a support group had been thwarted and forbidden in case they talked about their problems!

It is clear that talking about staff support is not the same as delivering it. There is much to do to translate the concept of good support into practice. It requires:

- Consistently good management and decision making
- Decisions to be communicated in a language which is universally understood
- Good communication channels, with clear and concise policy statements
- Evidence that policies are actually being carried out
- Use of teaching and in-service training opportunities
- Support networks in place with access for all
- Support for special needs where there is known pressure
- Debriefing facilities following exceptional trauma
- Good occupational health and counselling services, accessible to all
- Recognition of special needs where there are long term pressures
- Support during periods of uncertainty such as closures or threatened redundancy.

All of these offer better practical evidence of a caring culture and function where they are co-ordinated and recognised as staff support systems. An ethos of care can then evolve, enabling specific response to exceptional circumstances.

It is often said, 'We must make our staff *feel* valued'. But if the above services and conditions are seen to be in place, and are used, staff will *know* that they *are* valued and that this respect for their needs is a principle which is an integral part of the system, having equal consideration with other aspects of care. The organisation either values its staff or it does not consider this worth serious attention. Genuine care is always sincere and will be recognised.

An analogy to this is where an insecure person needs constant reassurance by being told that they are loved and accepted, whereas a secure person *knows* this is so, so needs less reassurance. They may appreciate being told, but the telling is not essential for the knowing. So what we are talking about is evidence of the attitudes and approach throughout the system that by its very nature says 'you are valuable', so they are constantly aware that this is so. It is noticeable that where staff are valued, this is evident throughout the system and is shown in the quality of team work and the level of quality care given, which in turn develops a sense of pride taken in the job and work standards. At a secondary level it shows in the attitude and personal appearance of staff and the way they relate to patients, relatives and each other.

A *philosophy for staff support* includes all the foregoing observations, which need to be refined and presented in a short, clear statement embodying what the particular organisation has to say. Constant revision is necessary during the discussion stages. It will embrace the balancing aspects of:

- Recognition of the range of needs to be taken into consideration
- Providing a network of services
- Creating a caring and supportive culture.

Inherent in this is a recognition that putting in a few support services in response to a crisis will only offer a kind of 'first aid' service. There needs to be a wider approach through a permanent network of services and supportive attitudes and culture. This built-in network will reduce the need for the heavy use of *crisis intervention*, because preventive aspects will be operating. Where a built-in system is well developed, it will reduce the possibility of severe damage to staff health and will minimise long term problems. It will be seen to improve staff confidence and overall efficiency.

Constantly caring for people in crisis is intensely demanding and the highest standards of safety and care are vital. The risk of error is increased where pressures are high. A caring staff resource is one of the largest and most essential resources in health services. These services are expected to meet the highest expectations of a public which is becoming more demanding and better informed all the time. The level of resources is apparent by looking at any budget. The rapid turnover and constant change of technological knowledge can be intensely demanding for staff who must be constantly alert in order to keep professionally competent to give required services to patients and families (Stoter 1995a) and so enhance recovery and rehabilitation.

The need to allocate resources for an efficient service is widely recognised for technology and servicing machinery, equipment and information technology. The time is now right to do the same for the labour force, but this will need an informed and careful approach to direct resources into the most efficient channels so that each component enhances the rest, and makes the most efficient use of available resources. This gives the rationale for preparing a policy for support and considering comprehensive proposals for a system. An informed approach is needed towards policy, plans, costs and benefits; these aspects will be discussed in the rest of this section.

Building on the evidence

Most of us can identify with the *experiences* described in the previous paragraphs and can recognise the importance of basing our policies on these factors. However, before managers invest resources in promoting any policy they will seek *hard facts* to justify expenditure on implementing a system. Until the 1990s the kind of hard facts or statistics they need to convince them have not been easy to select in order to justify proposals. (These issues are explained more fully in Chapter 9.)

The emerging picture

Early interest in this field began to attract attention with research in the 1960s into the origins and nature of stress and the individual's response (Menzies 1960a, b; Selye 1960; Revans 1962). The NASS review (Owen 1993) observed this trend and found that about 70% of publications over a period of ten years were concentrated on the nature, causes and effects of stress; about 10% focused on coping mechanisms, and about 10% were concerned with post-traumatic stress disorder. The remainder included a gradually increasing group of papers looking at costs and benefits of stress management, litigation and cultural change.

These proportions have varied only slightly since 1989, with a growing concern about the last three subjects mentioned. The number of studies in each group has quadrupled in the 1990s, and there has been a more sophisticated academic approach. The general trend is towards well-structured research on the nature and origins of stress, often focused on a particular profession or occupation. The interest in organisational stress leading to stress management in the workplace, has been much more prevalent in the 1990s.

Earliest attempts to deal with stress in health care were concentrated on individual coping mechanisms. Only in recent years has there been a move towards management concerns with organisational aspects. This is evident in the introduction of the 'Health at Work in the NHS Campaign' in the 1990s and positive moves to address organisational stress. Good research encouraged support for these aspects of concern particularly the work of Cooper and others of the University of Manchester Institute of Science and Technology (UMIST). There followed a growing tendency for organisations to mount short courses in stress management or to send individual staff members on one-day courses, but with no arrangements for follow-up in the practical situation. There is little evidence that these practices were worthwhile in reducing stress levels and the accompanying ill effects.

New evidence

A new and interesting trend is emerging from the thorough research carried out by the University of Manchester Institute of Science and Technology (UMIST), which indicates the most effective approaches to this widely recognised problem, in industry or large organisations such as the National Health Service. Emerging evidence supports many observations made from experience, that where organisations work with individuals in full participation there is a much more effective response, with positive reduction in the undesirable effects of stress imbalance (Cartwright 1996; Cooper et al. 1996).

These findings support observations made by those with long experience in the practice of staff support. This is the basis for the practical suggestions set out in this section of the book. A great strength lies in the process of empowering the individual to recognise their contribution as valuable and important, and to work together with the organisation to find and implement the most effective approaches to local needs. The value of a systematic or holistic approach becomes apparent, together with the recognition of the importance of a support *culture* as the fabric which holds the various parts together, providing and uniting the whole organisation in promoting a caring ethos.

Preparing a staff support policy

Understanding the nature of staff support and the supporting philosophy, together with evidence from research, are all part of the preparation for formulating a staff support policy and strategic plan of action. A *policy* is a statement agreed by the employers and staff based on the philosophy of the organisation, and on the aims and purpose of staff support which are the basis for future action. Many employers now publish a policy statement, together with a charter which embodies their ideals, standards and purposes.

Wide ranging evidence and information is needed as a foundation for formulating a policy. The first question many managers will ask when looking at this issue is, 'How much will it cost?'. There is no standard answer to this question because most statistics are applicable only to particular situations and therefore cannot be applied generally. It also depends on the nature of the provision required. Further detailed discussion on costs is given in Chapter 9, and also in a paper by NASS (1992a). The real question that should be asked is, 'What will it cost if I do *not* put in a good staff support system?'. To answer this, issues such as absenteeism, sickness rates, staff turnover (Revans 1962) and staff performance must all be balanced against any costs involved. Counselling services can be useful but can be expensive too unless they are properly backed up by preventive principles. A policy statement needs to include possible preventive measures and the identification of existing resources. A more complicated assessment of needs is then made, which takes time.

An important first move is to involve representatives of any existing services offering other aspects of staff support such as:

- Occupational health services
- Chaplaincy dept staff
- Education departments
- Management and personnel staff
- Staff responsible for communications
- Counselling service
- Peer support groups
- In service training opportunities
- Union representatives
- Staff responsible for communication structures or working environment.

Active participation from these staff will ensure the backing of all departments and will give an accurate picture of what is already being done and the most vulnerable areas which should be targeted first and receive priority finance.

Any policy statement must set out principles and aims leading to specific goals that are realistic within a given period. This involves each employee in identifying a personal contribution which can be made in their own workplace. By contributing to a policy statement they will feel part of the system and will be supportive to further plans. The policy will have a mission statement which will be the foundation for developing a strategic plan setting out priorities and goals. The *process* of preparing a staff support policy is discussed in the remaining chapters of this section. Working through this process, involving key staff and using participative methods, will enable priorities to be identified and targeted accurately and in a way which meets *local* needs. The NASS Charter for Staff Support (NASS 1992b) sets out some general guidelines for policy makers which have been found useful by many trusts and other employers as they were established by a group already experienced in this area. It has now been well tried and remains a useful and comprehensive guide. These are a few examples of the principles suggested:

- Health care staff have the right to be valued
- Staff need help to recognise and acknowledge needs
- Each health authority should be responsible for setting a policy
- This policy should be accessible to all staff
- They must all have access to the services
- They should have access to appropriate debriefing facilities when needed
- Staff are entitled to a good working environment
- Managers also have needs and rights
- All rights bring responsibilities with them.

It is often forgotten that managers also have needs and are entitled to loyalty and support from staff.

The caring culture

Any cultural environment inevitably influences attitudes and practices. As already mentioned, carers find it difficult to recognise and accommodate their own needs, but traditions are changing and the approach to staff care is seen to need the same structured consideration as is given to patient care.

Staff need encouraging to take responsibility for their own care and not to view it just as a management responsibility. The contribution from pressures outside work – from the home and family – are also being given more recognition. Many firms today offer counselling for staff who have family problems or have had a recent bereavement. The OPUS report notes:

> '... it is simplistic to think of health care staff solely as victims of organisational stress ... we perpetuate some of the dysfunctional organisational arrangements which surround us ... and are also subject to pressures outside our control.' (Health at Work in the NHS 1995a)

This report acknowledges the range of pressures affecting staff at work and offers an intervention model with useful guidelines for planners.

It is essential to maintain dialogue between managers and staff throughout planning and negotiations, to prevent assumptions being made and unrealistic plans being formed which could cause friction later.

The process

Setting up a staff support system is *a process* starting with the formulation of a *policy*, through careful *assessment* and *consultation*, taking all the *evidence* into consideration. Once the policy is agreed it has to be set out, *communicated*, maintained and frequently *reviewed* and *revised* to meet the ever changing working conditions. The participants also need to be kept in touch with the process.

A key factor to success is maintaining a good, current assessment of needs and ensuring that they are met. The next chapter will show a way of achieving this and building it into an active policy.

Key points

(1) The nature of staff support needs clarification and definition.
(2) A clear policy needs to be formulated based on the philosophy of the organisation.
(3) Preparation of the policy needs to involve active participants and to take account of local needs.
(4) Support is an ongoing process that needs to be maintained, and strategies need to be revised.

Exercise

(5.1) Write down a few preliminary thoughts on a philosophy for staff support for your organisation or department. Keep these for future reference after you have read the next few chapters.

Chapter 6

The Process of Creating a Caring Culture

Dealing with a complex range of variables is always easier if attention is given to each specific part of the process as bite sized pieces. This information is then brought back into the context of the whole framework. In this way it is easier to build up an accurate picture covering all areas. As Toffler showed in his far-sighted work in 1970, success is more likely with this approach and with goals that are attainable, so bringing a sense of achievement.

For the framework we can use the three criteria suggested by Biley (1989):

- *intrapersonal* – dealing with factors within or relating to the individual
- *interpersonal* – dealing with factors within or relating to groups or teams
- *extrapersonal* – dealing with aspects of the wider organisational setting external to the individual and groups.

Exploration within these three areas helps identify needs and appropriate staff support provision, and is fundamental to the building in of supportive mechanisms. These are set in the context of the professional ethos and culture. The later chapters look at this and take an integrated view of the overall picture. It sounds a complicated approach but in fact this *awareness* of the total situation becomes part of any consideration of this subject and enhances any decisions made.

The first step, once the origins of pressures have been established, is to identify the needs and to sort out priorities. The essential *preventive* measure, before making decisions about the kind of support system needed, is to decide:

- Which stressors can be eliminated
- Which stressors can be limited or reduced
- Which stressors have to be accepted and therefore need built-in support mechanisms.

The individual approach

All groups or organisational teams are made up of individuals at different levels of responsibility. Individuals in health care, however, are all influenced by a kind of 'collective confusion' due to the fact that traditional approaches to care tend to reinforce the difficulty in seeing themselves as ordinary humans. Staff have the same basic needs for care and understanding as patients, and they need to recognise this fact.

There is also a tendency for staff to expect management to provide all staff support, but this ignores the fact that each person has a responsibility for their own wellbeing and actions.

Recognition and identification

Recognition of personal need is therefore the place to begin – developing a capacity to see oneself as being as vulnerable as any other human. Sometimes the pressures arise from a personal lifestyle that can be modified to remove some unnecessary demands on time or by setting realistic and acceptable priorities. Fighting against internal dissatisfaction can be exhausting. Constant failure to achieve results brings tiredness and so decreases the ability to make decisions and evaluate progress, which in turn brings further dissatisfaction, and so the downward spiral of pressures begins.

Recognition is being able to identify needs at all levels and to differentiate needs from wants (Bradshaw 1972). This applies at all three levels – managerial, team and individual – and is equally true for society, work and personal situations.

A patient visits his doctor complaining of excessive tiredness and the doctor asks him what he is doing at present. After describing a highly demanding lifestyle he complains of not sleeping, of lack of energy and general fatigue. After listening, the doctor asks him what he can expect if he is burning the candle at both ends. The patient replies, 'I didn't come here to be told what I already know, I came here to get some more tallow!'. Often we attempt to ask for more tallow when we know it is not available; that is a 'want' and not a 'need'.

Wants cannot necessarily be met and the damaging effects exhaust the resources available. This humiliates the individual and sets up a certainty of failure and a negative round of pressures. It is thus important to be realistic in identifying needs in the light of assessment of the resources available, particularly resources of time, skills, and access to support.

This is all about empowerment of the person, group or organisation. For example, when *attainable goals* are set it creates empowerment, bringing a sense of having control of the situation and control of one's life within the organisation. Absence of this control creates a sense of helplessness and powerlessness and creates disablement of the person or organisation, leading to frustration and potential failure.

Identifying the needs of the individual is a difficult process which includes things like:

- Assessing the history
- Recognising achievements and failures
- Recognising the reasons for these successes or failures
- Looking at skill levels, abilities and pressure points
- Examining personal pressures and internal conflicts
- Examining pressures from others and from the organisational environment.

It requires analysis within oneself and with others to get cross references leading to conclusions that avoid history repeating itself. Sadly people often repeat the same failures over and over again.

'Who am I then? Tell me that first and then if I like being that person, I'll come up.
If not, I'll stay here until I'm someone else.'

Lewis Carroll: *Alice in Wonderland*

Here it will be useful to refer back to any personal stress levels which emerged by using the check list in Chapter 3.

One of the greatest lessons of history is that we never learn from history, so we must ensure that we do not reinvent the treadmill because we have neglected to analyse things effectively in the individual, the group and the organisation. The starting point must always be to analyse our *needs*.

It is useful to *examine oneself* for personal strengths and to itemise resources available, and where there is a shortfall to find ways of compensating. This can often be done by interaction between individuals in the group, creating new ideas and approaches.

Recognising the need for support and seeking it is a sign of strength and maturity rather than a failure to cope.

- It requires willpower and determination to adapt
- It involves wisdom
- It involves clarity of thought
- It requires a strategy for setting goals for change and meeting them
- It requires appropriate use of all the resources available
- It requires recognition of strengths, weaknesses and limitations.

There are times when goals must be reset to make them attainable and this is a way of removing some stressors. The objectives can always be extended or readjusted later. An important criterion for success is to be able to see that the way forward is feasible. Where failure is expected, it can be guaranteed. Where the goal is achievable, there is a high chance that it will be reached. Unrealistic goals are disabling, and facing them can paralyse the person, the team or the whole organisation. Reviewing and resetting goals on a regular basis in response to a changing situation is essential. It is vital to have a long term vision but within that to set achievable stepping stones, identifying 'bite sized' projects, and building on their success within an overall programme.

A feeling of failure often isolates because of the guilt and fear of acknowledging it. The fear of consequences and ultimately of job loss is always there. It is also about loss of self respect, perceived loss of status and value in the eyes of colleagues and managers, and ultimately loss of the approval of the organisation and its leaders.

A proper analysis of these needs will assist the action planned in:

- Setting attainable goals
- Ensuring resources are available to meet those goals

- Identifying the particular needs for support, for personal help from the group and organisation
- Keeping a receptive mind to the process of analysis, reappraisal and evaluation
- Keeping alert to changing support needs
- Maintaining a clarity of thought and vision.

The basic framework used in Figs 3.1, 3.2 and 3.3 is repeated in Figs 6.1 and 6.2 under different headings and so is seen from different perspectives.

Recognition of needs in the team

The team is made up of individuals, all of whom ideally will have been through this process of analysing needs. A well functioning team is a group of individuals valuing each other. If it is simply seen as a sum of individual contributions, there is no recognition of the value of teams at all. The value and strength of the team are created because the team is greater than the sum of the individual contributions: the values, skills and abilities of each individual are welded together into a compendium greater than that which a group of isolated individuals could produce. The good team does not rely simply on the strength of the leader, but its quality is demonstrated by the ability and achievements of the group as a whole, and its ability to produce desired results.

A good team well led enhances the performance of each member beyond what they bring to the group, because of what is received from others in the face to face interaction. A poor team under-performs, for where there is poor integration there will be disharmony and a lack of confidence in the leadership and each other. This affects the value of the performance of each individual and of the team.

The team needs to set its own realistic goals, using the strengths that each individual brings to the group. It allows for analysis of strengths and weaknesses and builds all this into the kind of positive experience which is creative and enables areas of weakness to be improved. That *creative element* is vital for group performance and is the 'extra' that a group can achieve beyond a collection of individual contributions. These principles apply within the organisation too.

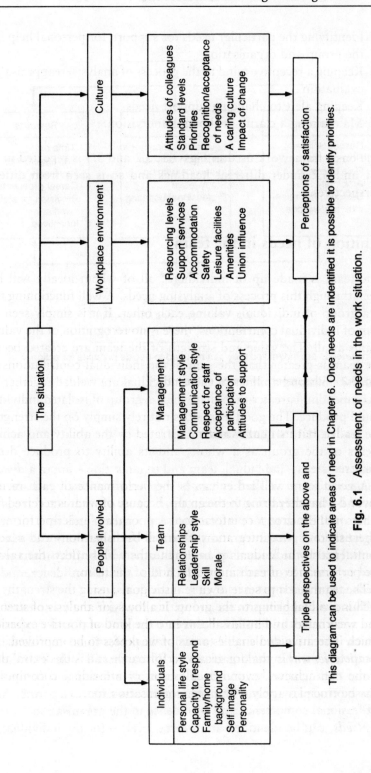

Fig. 6.1 Assessment of needs in the work situation.

This diagram can be used to indicate areas of need in Chapter 6. Once needs are indentified it is possible to identify priorities.

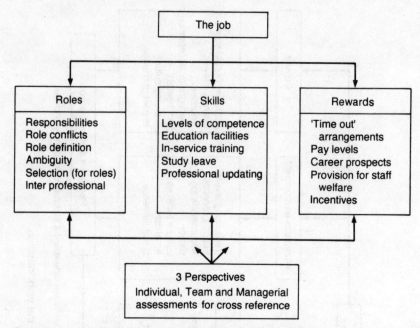

Once needs are indentified they can be used to decide priorities for action.

Fig. 6.2   Assessment of needs of the job.

Needs within the organisation

All three areas – individual, team and organisation – are in a *dynamic relationship* and while they can be explored separately, all are influenced by the interaction between them. So as the individual feeds into the group, the group's performance and quality feeds into the whole organisational structure and influences the organisational management. Healthy individuals in healthy teams with healthy management lead to a healthy organisation which has overall confidence, and this feeds into the competence of each individual area.

This is a complex process and within the NHS the complexity may be exacerbated by tensions between organisational and professional issues. The individuals need to maintain professional confidence and competence within the organisation. Where there is lack of confidence in the organisation, efficiency is inevitably affected and competence may be eroded over time. The need for success requires a partnership of professional competence and confidence in the organisation.

Needs, can be identified at all three levels – for the individual, the team and the organisation. In the healthy organisation objectives that are set will interrelate. Objectives, however, may be set by others outside the organisation, which may create conflict when clarity of objectives and the setting of realistic goals are critical in enabling good performance. The organisation is involved in removing excessive stressors, by naming realistic goals. Where the organisation is taking this kind of positive approach, basics like stress related illness, sickness rates and high staff turnover will be reduced. All these have an impact on the financial soundness of the organisation. The appearance of noticeable changes demonstrates that staff support works.

Recognition of need and the identification of the origins of excessive pressures are the first important steps in the process of meeting needs and providing support. Once stressors are identified, consider which can be limited or removed. For example, boredom for the individual or poor communications within a group can either be corrected or at least can be improved so that there is a better balance.

Assessment of need

Chapter 3 discussed assessment of need and its importance as an essential prerequisite for an action plan for staff support. But this is a complex procedure which can vary from a sophisticated research project involving meticulous scientific methods to a basic stress check carried out by students doing a small project for a diploma. Much energy is expended on questionnaires and attempts to measure stress levels, but research experts agree on the difficulties of producing accurate results (Hingley & Marks 1991).

One observation emerging from the NASS Literature Review (Owen 1993) relates to the rapid growth in the last few years of scientific publications with a wide approach and variety of methodologies illustrating many facets of the stressors involved in health care. However this varied approach makes it difficult to draw conclusions or make useful generalisations. The Review also highlights the fact that many of these studies are descriptive and analytic, emphasis the negative side of stress. There are few attempts to offer solutions or suggest positive approaches to staff support, until very recently. There is now a developing trend to address the problem by stress management programmes.

We must not fail to recognise the encouraging growth of good quality research material and studies on specific aspects appearing each year since 1990; neither must we underestimate the value of descriptive and evaluative studies, and audits on smaller scale projects. These studies all offer a contribution, but we need to be realistic in recognising the lack of a standardised assessment tool.

There are many good sources of literature on how assessment should be carried out (Health at Work in the NHS 1995a,b). It helps to consult an expert in a related field or someone with research experience, or experience in monitoring and audits, if the results are to be worthwhile. This is vital when preparing questionnaires, as badly worded or loaded questions can produce biased or inaccurate answers.

Factual evidence

Statistics on:
- Absenteeism
  — identifying excessives
  — monitoring changes
  — comparing with local and national standards
- Sickness levels (beware of distortions here)
  — monitoring levels
  — comparisons between departments, hospitals or
  — nature of

Quality assurance
- Using agreed criteria
- Measuring achievements, production, satisfaction

Morale
- Observation using different perspectives

Self-assessment
- Useful for monitoring stress levels
  — personal
  — workplace
  — professional

Using external professionals
- Research techniques

Fig. 6.3 Methods of assessing needs of staff support systems.

The investigator needs to ask himself several key questions:

- What is the purpose of this exercise?
- Is it to find information for producing an action plan?
- Is it to make comparisons with other national studies?
- Is it to compare with previous studies in this same area?
- What else has been done in this field?

The answers to these questions will guide the choice of tools to be used, the kind of questions to ask and who the respondents will be.

Figure 6.3 gives an overall perspective on the kind of tool which can be used for assessing needs. This will contribute to the overall approach to establishing a staff support strategy, which will include the following stages:

(1) Identification and location of pressures
(2) Assessment of needs throughout the system
(3) Listing of priorities – areas, locality, situations etc.
(4) Resources already available
(5) Plan for action – short term and longer term
(6) Setting up a monitoring–review process.

Figures 6.1 and 6.2 set out a framework for assessment covering the main areas and going on to identify priorities. This links with suggestions elsewhere in this text, such as identification of resources, and should be co-ordinated to formulate a plan of action for staff support.

Key points

(1) A useful framework to use in the staff support process is based on identifying needs for the individual, the team and the organisation.
(2) Preventive measures can be taken where pressures can be eliminated, reduced, or dealt with.
(3) The individual needs to recognise and take responsibility for personal needs, and develop strengths.
(4) Team needs must be recognised and met if the team is to function well.
(5) Organisational needs will vary in different settings.

(6) Needs must be properly assessed; models and a suggested tool for assessment are offered.

Exercises

(6.1) Write down what you consider to be your own personal pressures at this time. Then identify which pressures you think could be removed or limited in terms of damaging effects.

(6.2) Now write down some of your strengths which could be developed creatively.

Chapter 7

The Process – Personal Responsibilities and Peer Support

'The symphony needs each note
The book needs each word
The house needs each brick
The ocean needs each drop of water
The harvest needs each reaper
The whole of humanity needs you
as and where you are
    You are unique
No one can take your place
Begin now – why are you waiting.'

Michel Quoist: *The Breath of Love*

Support and care for the individual

Taking responsibility for one's own wellbeing means taking care in all aspects of life, including personal, social and working aspects. One obvious and important feature to assess is use of time. Time tends to be spent on areas considered to be important and is therefore a statement of priority; aspects that are not considered important tend to be left out. Some people who neglect one area of their lives often tend to become neglectful in other areas too. Others may give obsessive attention to one aspect at the cost of others. The very nature of a rounded individual is to be a balanced person. To perform effectively there needs to be fitness of mind, body and spirit, and care is needed to develop in all these areas for a rounded personality and to be fit. The overall principle is that energy levels are affected considerably by the level of care taken to maintain a balance and quality of life, physical, mental and spiritual. Balance is about keeping a freshness of outlook, variety of life and time for recreation, all of which maintain a zest for living, which pervades all aspects of life.

So the personal element in self care is vital. Having the back-up of friends and colleagues to share interests, to enjoy mutual exchange of ideas and listen is vital. It is important to know when to seek more professional support and help, and to know who to turn to when professional or counselling help is needed. One of the most difficult decisions is to know when to stop pushing oneself, and to say 'I need some time out, I need some space to myself', or learning to say, 'no, I cannot take on any more'. This is especially difficult where it appears to leave patients or clients unattended. Those kinds of decisions sometimes have to be made in self defence and in order to function efficiently, particularly where meticulous skill or precision decision making is required. All this is essential to good personal resourcing, for which each individual holds considerable responsibility.

Practical ways of coping

There is much good advice about 'stress management and self help' in various leaflets and articles in professional journals. Many of these can be informative and helpful for the interested individual and some can be found in the reading list at the end of this book. A helpful booklet is published by the Health Education Authority (Woodham 1995). This and many similar sources will remind readers of the signs of excessive stress and provide check lists and suggestions for personal management (see also Chapter 3). Note particularly the importance of recognising early symptoms and taking immediate action. Much can be done at this stage by individuals taking personal responsibility for their own lives. This calls for:

- Recognition of the signs of imbalance at an early stage
- Knowing one's personal strengths and weaknesses
- Identifying the sources of pressures and eliminating them where possible
- Taking responsible action where pressure is inevitable
- Reviewing one's lifestyle
- Seeking help when the pressures become excessive.

There are many ways in which changes in lifestyle can help, for example:

- Careful planning of priorities, and learning to say 'no' when appropriate

- Finding and using friends or family support where available
- Planning the use of time – taking time out for proper relaxation
- Making use of any leisure breaks and facilities available at work
- Making good use of support services at work.

In the longer term this may involve assessing one's job satisfaction and fulfilment or considering a change in career paths, especially if there are clashes between home commitments and work demands. This may be difficult to achieve in today's climate. It may be that the individual feels helpless to take personal control of the situation, or even has lost the ability to assess things logically. This is when it is important to seek outside help and make use of other expertise.

> 'The great art of riding as I was saying, is to keep your balance – "like this you know". Here he let go of the bridle and stretched out both his arms to show Alice what he meant, and this time he fell flat on his back.'

> Lewis Carroll: *Alice Through the Looking Glass*

There are many alternative steps that can be taken once the person recognises the need for help. It is important to have a physical health check, to deal with any physical problems. Some immediate relief can be found through some kind of relaxation therapy, such as music, reading, walking when opportunity permits, talking with friends or family when they can listen and enlisting their practical support. Increasingly there are facilities in the workplace, such as aromatherapy or reflexology treatment, relaxation or meditation groups. There may be exercise facilities, or simply the rest room, chapel or some other place where peace and quiet can be found, to unwind. Supportive managers will help in identifying and facilitating this.

These are examples of how individuals can find help and take responsibility for their own wellbeing, but there are times when it takes someone else to recognise a cry for help or the need for more professional help. This help may be provided in the form of a support group, either within the workplace or outside, or in the occupational health service, the chaplaincy or in a counselling service.

Sometimes further action may be needed, when an individual is advised to take a break from work. This should not be regarded as a failure to cope, but rather an opportunity for assessment and personal development, and often can lead to greater maturity in the individual who may become more understanding and sensitive to their own and others needs. Individual help from a professional counsellor may be necessary for a while.

Team or group resources

All individuals belong to groups and here we consider the groups within the health care workplace, their need for support, and their role in providing support for group members.

The first step is for each member of a group to be careful of others in the same way that they care for themselves. To start 'listening' to what is being said or indicated, whether the needs are expressed openly or become apparent in some kind of behaviour, is a beginning. All this is inherent in valuing others in the team, in recognising their needs, whether spoken or silently expressed, and in learning how to identify and note specific pressures common to all, or those that affect certain individuals. Work pressures are usually easily spotted but it is less obvious when the pressures come from some other aspects of an individual's life. *Sensitivity* to others' needs can be cultivated within a group.

> A student nurse who attended her mother's funeral on Friday afternoon, returned to work on Monday morning. The first task she was given was to go and attend to the needs of a family whose relative had just died and to deal with the necessary procedures for the patient and family. After a short time she returned in tears to say she could not continue to deal with the situation adequately as her own grief was too fresh. She was sent off duty and told if she could not manage her own bereavement and act professionally she should not be in nursing at all! That nurse eventually completed her course and became an extremely sensitive and caring practitioner, but she could so easily have acted on the advice to 'get out' and her profession would have lost an excellent nurse and many patients would have been deprived of someone who had a wealth of understanding and quality of care to give.

Acceptance of vulnerability is part of the process of receiving support and is essential to knowing how to offer support.

Peer support

Peer support covers both formal and informal support mechanisms. It is important to recognise the opportunities that exist within the system already and to be alive to the possibilities of bringing in new systems. An accurate analysis of what is going on is essential, which should not be an emotional appraisal but a realistic assessment of what is happening. For example, it is only too easy to say 'we get absolutely no support', which may be quite untrue. Team members may be giving very active support for much of the time, and this must be recognised and enhanced.

At times there can be almost a sense of pride in saying 'I get no support', which can mean assumptions are being made and different interpretations are being put on what is 'support'. It is often said that 'nobody cares' about staff needs, when a great deal of care is actually given, and this statement can be a reflection of the individual's feelings of frustration and helplessness at being unable to see ways of changing a situation or maintaining it acceptably.

Often what is needed is for someone to listen actively at the time of an incident, or soon after. The health staff involved with the King's Cross fire disaster were reported as saying that their most valuable form of support was through colleagues or other people who would just listen to them and let them talk (Rosser 1991). This is a valuable but often unrecognised form of support which requires colleagues to recognise the importance of listening and to recognise the signs that someone needs to talk or to express grief, bewilderment, anger or shock. Peer support is therefore a valuable element, so often undervalued or overlooked.

After a traumatic episode staff can be heard to say that they had no support, because the only form of support recognised is a formal debriefing session, or emergency counselling service. Often the really effective support is the immediate listening and practical recognition given at the scene. Unless a resource is 'labelled' in some way, its value may fail to be recognised or be given status within the system.

For an individual or team member to say 'I get no support' may be a statement about that person, indicating a personal unwillingness or inability to accept what is offered in its simplest form. Some people derive status from a martyr syndrome within which it is essential not to receive any care or support in order to be able to say, 'I spend my life giving care to others but no one cares about me'. The peer group can help each member of the team to recognise the understanding, care and support which they can give to one another, by recognising the common areas of need and also the needs or problems specific to individuals. The peer group can also encourage members to accept help from within the group and to seek outside help where appropriate. The giving of care is an act of valuing. Identifying the support and value that is already in place is a foundation stone for building upon. The support will be built and endorsed in a way that is appropriate for the team and its members, and can thus be an aid to enhance the effectiveness of the team.

The support may mean identifying a member of the team who has shown particular sensitivity or skills, and encouraging that person to develop and use those skills for the benefit of the team. It may mean identifying particular occasions when the team members meet for discussion or debriefing, and using these more effectively. It may mean particular in-service training or self-development for some members, to help them to recognise personal needs and the needs of colleagues who need particular support, care and encouragement, or to identify those whose personal relationships need extra care.

Where individuals in a team, or team leaders, have a feel for those approaches, they can be a catalyst within that team to enhance a caring environment and a sensitivity to need.

Identification of different kinds of groups

In addition to the general team ethos of caring, there may be other informal or formal oppportunities for support which can contribute, providing the contribution is recognised and built upon. Informal networks are found in situations such as ward meetings or tea breaks, where there are opportunities to look at the roles of individuals and reflect on feelings and needs, to value individuals, so giving continuous informal support.

Thus the basic foundation of a caring ethos within the team is important if it is to be effective to the group as a whole. Without it the group is likely to be less effective than it could be.

There are a number of informal groups already in existence within the system, within different professions, groups of friends and peers; sometimes they have existed for a long time, sometimes they happen for a short period only. Team support is constantly evolving. The team will contain long-stay members and other members who move in and out more frequently. It is important that members learn to value one another and share their skills, so that they can think and plan and take action together. Groups do not become teams by just throwing individuals together. Members need to work together, to practise together and to be together for a while. To have a collection of skilled and experienced individuals does not necessarily mean they will form a good team.

Another informal element which can be strengthening to the team is courtesy and consideration for one another, backed up by the more formal aspect of good communication both written and verbal. There is also the aspect of training and developing skills together and learning to function as a group, trusting one another and valuing each other's skills, ideas, hopes, fears and achievements.

Within a team it is important to allow opportunities to:

- Reflect on what is happening
- Reflect how care is being delivered
- Allow for reassessment of situations
- Allow the team to reconsider its strategy
- Facilitate the most effective use of each person.

Quite small changes can result in improvements in the effectiveness of the team and can influence the quality of care and job satisfaction.

An example of a small change resulting in a major improvement was the removal of a door and wall on a particular ward. This allowed the nurses' station to be moved, which in turn allowed the nursing practice to change. This benefited patients and staff. The action arose out of a ward meeting to address issues of staff morale.

So it is important to use existing groups such as team meetings and case conferences for informal support. Members learn to understand each other's attitudes and this can influence the ethos of care between meetings.

Specific support groups come into being for a variety of reasons. Examples can be seen of groups with a common interest and need, such as bereaved relatives, people who have cancer, parents who have lost children, or individuals who have been involved in a major incident. In all these groups there is a common interest and a common need. It is a powerful stressor to be exposed to demands one is not really prepared to meet, both for members of the group and for the person leading it. Leading these groups demands much sensitivity, fairness and the ability to encourage participation and to be nondirective. Facilitating is a better word to use than leading. Part of the facilitator's task is to 'make it safe' for the participants. Hence, it is important to agree on the basic guidelines and rules for the group, making sure that everyone is conversant with and prepared to accept the rules.

To facilitate a group needs a level of maturity and the ability to allow the agenda to be set by the group rather than the facilitator, and to allow exploration of questions which have no answers. At the same time there is a danger that the group could become a 'whinge' group and use the situation to 'take one another down', so they might go out feeling worse than when they came in. It is important to look for ways of relieving the pressures identified and of leaving the group meeting on a positive note but one based on reality.

In the early stages it is often valuable to have an external facilitator to give some focus and structure to the group and to help in establishing ground rules.

Setting up formal group support

Preparation and assessment

Clarification of some important issues is a prerequisite to establishing a successful support group. The first question is what kind of support group is needed, and whether it is feasible. It may be:

- A *small peer group* in your own unit to meet specific needs in the short or longer term
- A *facilitator led group* confined to your own team or including a range of staff from different units
- A *therapist led group* to concentrate on personal development or in-depth work, using therapeutic processes
- A *group providing facilities* for relaxation techniques, reflexology, aromatherapy or other forms of alternative therapy.

There are many variations on this theme and within the above framework there are other issues to consider about the *kind of process* most appropriate for the group. It may be:

- A *problem solving* group, e.g. in a local situation to resolve problems particular to that group

- An *action learning* group, e.g. this may be useful in a period of innovation or change to provide feedback on progress
- A *training group* to develop specific skills in self assertiveness, or sensitivity development for personal needs or for the team
- A group offering *de-briefing and support* following a particular crisis or major disaster.

Although *local needs* are of prime consideration, choices may to some extent depend on *resources* or expertise available. If there is no specialist leadership available it may be possible to enlist some local support for an in-house venture. Access to some form of supervision for the facilitator is important, to give personal support and to help if the group develops 'negative' attitudes or becomes stuck, which can have a downward spiral effect and can lead to deep emotional conflicts within the group.

The next consideration concerns the *resources* needed. This includes such basic questions as:

- What *managerial support* do you have?
- Are there any *financial resources* available?
- Do you have *access to an experienced facilitator*, or can you pay for someone outside your organisation?
- Do you have colleagues with *training and experience in leading* such groups?
- What kind of *accommodation* is available for your use and where is it?
- Is there someone willing to take *responsibility for administrative aspects* of running such a group?

There are other points to consider such as frequency and length of meetings, number of sessions planned, number of members in any one session, and whether the group is a closed group or whether others may join.

One of the first points to establish when the group meets is the aim and purpose of the group. *Ground rules* are essential for any successful group and include agreement on *all* the above points, particularly:

- Attendance – must it be every meeting? What do you do about absenteeism?
- The policy about members joining
- Confidentiality within the group. Members need to have assurance

that everything said within the group is confidential and can only be taken out of the group with the agreement of all the members.

Reappraisal and revision of these ground rules may be necessary from time to time, also reappraisal and evaluation of the group on a regular basis.

The quality of leadership is important for success in a group and an experienced leader is clearly advisable, although not always available. Sometimes groups can function adequately without a leader, apart from administrative aspects. Qualities desirable for leading a group include good listening and interpretive skills and sensitivity.

Evidence of the effectiveness of support groups

There is often an assumption that 'support groups are a good thing and therefore we need one', but this may not always be the case. The evidence is not conclusive and sometimes appears contradictory. Many authors have presented evidence making a good case for setting up a support group. Alexander *et al.* (1993) says such groups help one to realise one is not alone in a predicament and that one's feelings, fears and reactions are shared by others. This brings mutual support and good support enables professionals to function more effectively (Farrell 1992). It cannot be assumed that to get together once a week is automatically therapeutic. A group may well develop into a ritual of its own and become a source of stress itself, especially if attendance is compulsory.

One writer suggests there is a *possible hazard* in that support groups may lead to staff accepting less than ideal working situations as 'they help people to tolerate the intolerable' (Harvey 1992). Alternatively the group could become an agent for change, to improve these conditions as the members become less stressed and are more able to think creatively.

One occasion when it is certain that support groups will make an important contribution to staff wellbeing is in the event of a major incident or disaster, when some kind of debriefing and ongoing support has been clearly shown to be of use (Owen 1990).

Albrecht and Adelman (1984) concluded from their literature review that support groups could meet needs for venting feelings, providing reassurance and improving communication skills. They can also reduce uncertainty and give increased confidence, and provide resources and companionship, so aiding recovery where appropriate (Spinks & Bowering 1990).

Tschudin (1988) points out that groups offer anonymity in dealing with personal and work related problems, enabling members to deal more effectively with situations. Members recognise a common vulnerability which enables them to discover how much they are able to give each other.

Rosenfeld and Richman's study (1987) was unable to demonstrate any significant reductions in stress levels following support groups, but important differences were found according to the type of group selected. Effectiveness of groups depends heavily on selecting the right type of group, and on the commitment of its members.

So there are many ways in which individuals can recognise needs for support and groups can help to provide it. They are a resource which can contribute to the system as a whole and, as the next chapter shows, they need recognition by those assessing the planning needs for the organisation.

Key points

(1) There are ways in which individuals can take responsibility for assessing their own needs and coping with pressures. They also need access to personal support at times.

(2) Groups can provide peer support for members and can be utilised to meet special needs.

(3) Where formal support groups are established, setting up and following ground rules will be essential for success.

Exercises

(7.1) Outline some of the pressure areas in your own lifestyle which could be prevented or limited.

(7.2) How do you cope with pressures in your own life? Identify some of your own ways of coping with them and also where you can go for help.

(7.3) What support groups can you identify in your own sphere of work? How do these contribute to easing pressure in the workplace? This exercise could be useful for a group discussion.

(7.4) How would you go about setting up a support group in your own unit or department?

Chapter 8

Organisation and Management – Systems and Service

The response to pressures from individuals and groups has been considered, so now the third perspective to explore is the management or organisational one. Silverman (1984) points out that the actions of participants are governed by their own personal definitions of the situation, and not that of any other observer. Therefore, we need to look at these different perspectives because all participants have different perceptions of a situation depending on their expectations. These in turn are affected by status, culture, professional attitudes and many other factors.

Early organisational theory tended to be based on a structural model, presenting a general view of a one-dimensional diagram rather like a large piece of engineering in terms of structures and systems, input and output, with a heavy concentration on management and control (Handy 1991). Currently more recognition is given to the importance of interaction between people, and the influences of culture, politics, networks and teamwork (Silverman 1984). The emphasis has shifted from control to power and from management to leadership. It is recognised today that to make any structure operational and to ensure efficient functioning, there are many factors which need consideration.

The culture of an organisation influences the way any staff support system operates. It includes *values, ideologies and expectations*, and *assumptions*, and it helps to maintain cohesiveness and order for the members (Handy 1991).

A vital aspect frequently overlooked is the human resource, a most important element if the whole process is to work efficiently. Human resources are infinitely variable and affected by many influences, in the workplace and outside, which affect performance. This makes selection, management and leadership styles, for example, vital ingredients of the whole process. Human nature is influenced by the prevailing culture, and by local working conditions or current events. Technical equipment, accommodation, location and financial resources are all major issues. Communication styles are also significant as an organisation is a dynamic entity full of life, with constant movement and interaction between the various parts.

Examples of this communication process can be seen in nature. If you watch a mature tree in full leaf you will notice that the leaves form intricate and artistic patterns, having a particular relationship to main branches, trunk and roots. When a slight breeze springs up the peripheral leaves all move in relationship to each other, the intricate patterns constantly changing, but the relationship with the branch remains stable within the overall structure, so contact with the roots is ensured. This example can provide much food for thought where the processes in an organisation are concerned. If a leaf or a branch gets separated from the trunk or badly damaged, performance is damaged and in some cases destroyed.

The more you think about this example the more it illustrates the importance of the human resource element of the organisation. It is a valuable resource that needs nurturing, needs care and respect itself, and is likely to 'expect' this or to look to the 'organisation' for that. Its expectations and requirements are influenced by current thought and the prevailing culture of the organisation and the outside world (see Chapters 10 and 11).

What is less often recognised is that the staff *themselves* are purveyors of culture; they communicate their own values and attitudes very quickly among each other (Bach 1972). They can perpetuate negative attitudes, or form a creative force *for* the organisation. The organisation or management working *with* the staff is much more powerfully creative and more likely to succeed.

The managerial role in an organisation

This chapter concentrates on some of the practical realities in setting up a staff support system, from the managerial perspective, and this involves both a process and the attitudes of the prevailing culture. Part of the managerial role is to provide the appropriate resources needed to establish the process, but part is about the cultural approach which permeates the whole organisation. In this sense the management can be seen as offering a role model, as an organisation's culture will reflect the managerial style as well as influencing it (Handy 1991).

The process – providing services

The first question most people ask is what managers can or should provide. This can mean a wide variety of services, many of which may already be in place and functioning well under different names, such as occupational health, chaplaincy, education, and others listed in Chapter 5. There are, however, additional provisions which indicate the way in which the staff are valued as a resource. These include ensuring the best possible systems for pay and reward, good disciplinary systems, and recognition of the rights and responsibilities of both employees and managers. The way these processes are set up can indicate a sense of fairness and recognition. Pay and reward systems are contentious areas so there must be fairness in making allocations, in allocating responsibility and in grading systems, duty rosters, arrangements for time out and various other processes where jealousy and resentment can be fostered and so lead to stressful relationships.

> A situation that sometimes arises and causes resentment is when a member of staff with specialist skills but a low grade is involved in transferring a patient from another similar unit, and finds the professional colleague transferring the patient has fewer qualifications and less experience and responsibility, but is allocated a higher grading. There are many similar instances which give rise to dissatisfaction and resentment.

It is not unknown for managers to set up an expensive counselling service and expand the occupational health provision, and assume that staff support has been adequately provided for, or alternatively to plead lack of resources, or even to terminate an existing provision because results are not apparent immediately.

Further reference will be made to ways in which the value of services can be maximised and costed (Chapter 9), as this is an important criterion for making a case for resource allocation (Channon *et al.* 1990). The value and performance of existing services can be increased by proper use and recognition of the support element inherent in the services, and by enhancing the skills of staff in key positions of leadership to equip them with listening skills and to recognise signs of pressure etc.

Ways and means – bringing together the supporting culture

Creating the right kind of cultural environment for a particular organisation can have effects far beyond staff support and can make the whole organisation run more smoothly. A caring environment is infectious and quickly picked up by all involved. It is communicable throughout the staff and once established it is passed on to patients, relatives and others using the organisation. It has a profound effect on newcomers and helps them to respond quickly and become part of a caring team. A caring attitude smoothes procedures at interview and attracts and retains good quality staff. It also creates conditions favourable for learning and creativity among staff, so improving the overall morale and performance of staff and providing quality care for patients.

The managers have an important part to play in all this and can act as a visual aid or role model. Those with greater responsibilities set the tone which encourages positive attitudes in the various units, teams of professionals and all individuals making up the organisation. This kind of cultural environment is created by having a caring attitude to staff in all policy making, in management style and attitudes, and by the staff perceiving this commitment. Some managers have greater input than others by virtue of their seniority.

> 'An organisation's culture is reflected in many ways and influences, not only its structure and managerial style, but also the way in which it conducts its business in the widest sense.'

> (Cartwright & Cooper 1994)

There are ways by which management can help the creation and nurturing of a caring attitude throughout the system, encouraging a committed workforce 'owning' that culture. This creates harmony, unity and good teamwork, encouraging mutual understanding and support between individuals, and avoiding the culture of fear, repression and divisiveness. This may sound a Utopian dream to some people but it is not impossible to feed these concepts into the process if recognition is given to the channels which can be utilised, including:

- *Routine communication* channels
- Utilisation of *skills*
- Working through educational *opportunities*
- *Fairness* in allocation and use of *resources*
- *Participation of the workforce.*

Communication channels need to be good and there must be two way

communication both up and down the line so that there are *opportunities* for staff to receive information and feed back their own ideas,
views and responses to management. This is often best done in a discussion forum where there is an opportunity to explore ideas and
debate some of the practical suggestions from staff involved at all
levels. That way a creative atmosphere is engendered and employees
feel part of the decision making process. Opportunities may be found
frequently in team meetings, professional meetings or specially con-
vened meetings, the main point being that that there is a freedom for
staff to join in and feel they can influence decisions, offer amendments
or even avert disasters. Freedom to express views will go a long way
towards eliminating stressful pressures in an organisation.

Establishing good two way *communications* is about openness and a
willingness to listen, and about clarifying difficult concepts. It is about
adaptation to and acceptance of various points of view, about sharing
purpose and planning. This all involves certain skills – *the skills* of
presentation with clarity and simplicity. It means taking complex and
profound subjects and introducing them in a way which can be
understood by staff, patients and relatives, and is accessible to all,
including the public in the wider perspective. Policy statements need to
be formed on a clearly thought through vision and purpose, showing
manageable objectives that can be achieved, again presented with
clarity and simplicity and freedom from jargon. This does not mean
'talking down' to people, but rather using short and clear statements
and avoiding jargon and the temptation to say too much.

Culture is *communicable* and one skill is to take every opportunity
to cultivate and communicate a sense of valuing the individual, not just
on paper but through attitudes like fairness and the recognition of
contributions made and what individuals can offer, and valuing and
utilising the teams as integral cogs in an organisation. Another key area
is in demonstrating that *resources* are utilised well and *fairly* dis-
tributed. Poor decisions made without consultation generate much
anxiety and ill feeling, as when computer systems were installed
without consultation in the erroneous belief that they would automatically enhance communications and save money. It is interesting to
note how many computer systems have had to be replaced quickly
because the wrong or an inadequate system has been installed. Good
monitoring and auditing can avoid some errors of this kind.

Most experts agree that research studies available at present are
inadequate as a basis for formulating intervention procedures, hence it
is difficult for management to base firm proposals on evidence (Cox

1993). There are some studies which give some indication for guidance, such as the OPUS report on organisational stress (Health at Work in the NHS 1996) which cites a study done in Sweden that demonstrated that where staff participated in interventions and the unions collaborated, the effects were markedly improved.

The OPUS study indicated that there were three stages for the intervention process:

(1)   Raising staff awareness of work-related stress and its causes
(2)   Discussing and clarifying the connections between individual and work-related stress with clarity and with a new vocabulary
(3)   Planning and implementing system solutions.

Use of *resources* can so easily become a contentious issue, when staff see what they feel is waste of resources in any form, for example when they see many apparently useless papers being circulated, which are immediately binned. Awarding priority in resource allocation is a measure of value attached to that service and can so easily be seen as unfair where not properly explained or where the decision has not been discussed. Pay and reward systems do need to reflect priorities as a whole, so allocation must be fair, and often this is not reflected in national or local settlements.

Recognition of the need for compassionate leave and time out, or flexible rotas allowing for particular living needs or accommodation, is important. More effective deals could be explored with trusts and local firms to enhance spending powers of staff. Bonus deals or extra leave are all about rewarding, by recognition, the commitment and consistent hard work of the staff . So *fairness* must be present and must be seen to exist in so many key issues of rights, responsibilities, allocation of resources, grading, pay and rewards and all aspects of policy making.

Educational opportunities are another area which is often underdeveloped and which presents many channels for encouraging understanding of human development, awareness and self assertion, together with an understanding of methods of preventing pressures and handling stressful situations. Often staff are offered good courses in these topics, only to find that they bear little relationship to reality and are not supported in principle in practical situations (Stoter 1991). Courses need to provide built-in opportunities for development in application if their full value is to be realised. It is possible for all students to have insights into the subject built into their initial courses and this can be followed up throughout training and during post graduate courses and in-service training. The key point, for the learning to be effective, is that there should be appreciation of the need for support, and opportunities to reflect on progress and on self development in wards and units. This means that unit managers and senior staff need to be aware of the kind of training given and to be able to build on it.

An effective and caring organisation is a learning organisation. There is opportunity for exploring new ideas and carrying them out in an atmosphere of acceptance and supportive participation, where managers approve, the team is involved, and the organisation becomes creative with improved performance. Here there is an opportunity to make good use of appropriate literature as part of the educational process.

Mix and match process

It is important for management to identify and specifically draw out the different needs, philosophies and services to be clarified and recognised as part of the process of providing staff support. Some aspects are more easily identified than others, and some resources may already be in place, offering a supportive service within their own remit. For example, occupational health services are now mandatory, although much depends on the way the service operates and its use within the organisation. Areas of significance relate to skills of the staff, location and provision of services, and how well they liaise with human resources departments, chaplaincy services and others.

How such services operate is important. For example, most chaplains now recognise their role in supporting staff as well as patients, and many staff in these departments have counselling skills as part of their qualifications. However, styles vary and as with all professions, there are good and bad practices. Much depends on the quality of communication between staff and management.

At the beginning of the Gulf War many hospitals were rushed into recognising the need for staff support provision and NASS had many calls requesting advice on setting up emergency provisions. One morning eight different calls for help were received from eight different professionals in

(Contd)

one large hospital. They were located in different departments or units and had all been asked to prepare plans for setting up an overall service. Each one had no idea that others had been approached with the same request or had any skills to offer. When it was suggested they got together, pooling their resources as a group, this was welcomed as an opportunity to establish a quality service at the minimum cost. They discovered that by working together as a team, communications all round were improved, skills were shared and an excellent co-ordinated service emerged which was the foundation for the comprehensive service that exists today.

Other similar examples have been experienced, revealing the importance of professionals working together and understanding and sharing the skills they have. Networking between different professionals and teams can be a very productive influential ingredient which is not commonly practised within organisations. Managers need to facilitate and encourage this process.

Questions for consideration

There are many questions to be asked to ensure this process is efficient in utilising all the valuable opportunities and resources. We need to know:

- Is there good access to support when needed on the spot?
- Are the services and their function well known to all staff?
- Where does support come from (e.g. colleagues or services)?
- Can all managers or leaders recognise the warning signs of excessive stress?
- How are they trained to deal with what they see?
- How are they prepared to be effective and sensitive in delivering the service?
- What reward mechanisms does the organisation offer?
- Are the various reward strategies known (e.g. time out when needed)?
- Is sufficient appreciation shown when staff have overcome difficult moments?
- Are records kept on reasons for sickness and absenteeism?
- How is absenteeism dealt with?

It can be seen from these questions that there is a range of factors involved in offering quality support to staff, which really need to be incorporated by management in daily practice. These factors need to be clarified and built into policy statements and reports when rights and responsibilities are considered.

There is a role for government departments, trusts and health boards and health commissions, as well as for purchasers and providers of services. It is common to find no mention of staff support in overall budgets, but for it to be devolved to training budgets, time out allocations and appointment processes.

Role of management in providing staff support

This chapter has set out a broad perspective on the role of managers in providing opportunity for reflection, in gaining insights into the process of providing support and in recognising the importance of attitudes. Cox (1993), in his exhaustive study on the literature available, concludes that there is very little conclusive evidence on the value of different approaches. He comments:

> 'More research and development is required in relation to the measurement of the experience of stress and the overall stress process. The inadequacy of single "one off" measures is widely recognised in the literature but despite this they continue to be used ...'

In this chapter the range of aspects has been thoroughly explored and attitudes are seen as an important part of the process and a vital ingredient of the system. In summary, the important elements for managers to consider are:

- The *process* of setting up a system, which is built on assessment of need in the light of resources available and the services which already exist and function well. This makes it possible to identify gaps in the services. A useful check list is given by O'Kell (1993).
- The *attitudes of a caring culture* which reflect the management approach throughout the organisation.

These elements in turn are dependent on others, such as a clear concise policy reflecting purpose and vision and conveyed through good communication systems. Other important issues relate to the use of skill and recognition of rights and responsibilities, and the good use of opportunities in team work and education.

Fairness in resource allocation is seen as a major element and so managers need to have accurate information. This underlines the importance of regular monitoring systems to record progress and reassess needs and priorities, and these are discussed in the next chapter.

Key points

(1) Organisational structures, management styles and human resources are all important aspects to be considered in the process of assessing needs and providing support.

(2) The culture of support also plays a part in devising ways and means.

(3) Communication channels, skills, opportunities, education and resources are all means to facilitate the process.

(4) The process of 'mix and match' is also a way to bring all facilities together when setting up a system.

Exercise

(8.1) How would you describe the cultural ethos in your department or organisation?

Chapter 9

Monitoring the Process – Costs, Audits and Action

Research, monitoring and evaluation

Research

Research is obviously integral to development of staff support and should aim to identify clearly what needs there are, what resources are already in place, how effective they are in operation and to what extent they are appreciated by users. Research may vary from very simple questionnaires to fully planned projects establishing an academic basis with properly validated work. At the most sophisticated level this may take a considerable time and proper funding, and may require the skills of a team of experts. The simple questionnaire can be used within the team in a particular area; this avoids the problem of one strong person imposing his/her view of need on others. There should be an opportunity for all members of staff in that particular area to respond in a carefully considered way to a range of questions. This method can be used by managers to carry out a comprehensive survey of all staff in a particular area, or to take a sample across the organisation and develop a cross referencing system.

An in-house approach clearly demands objectivity of the person carrying it out. It is useful to have an external researcher for the more formal and comprehensive exercises, as such a person has no internal interest or bias. Even a member of staff doing a simple questionnaire in the local work area will benefit from constructive advice and assistance from someone who has experience in preparing such questionnaires, to avoid the possibility of bias towards certain kinds of answers. Questionnaires should be prepared in such a way that the answers can easily be collated. A small pilot study is a helpful tool which can quickly provide an insight into the particular area.

When carrying out research of any kind relating to individuals' views on stress, there are many variables involved. If this is not realised answers are likely to be subjective and influenced by suggestion in the questions. This does not mean that findings of such studies are useless, but it does mean that the limitations must be recognised. There are many well validated, published studies on identification of the causes of stress in different professions (e.g. Cooper *et al.* 1990; Dewe 1991; Johnson 1991; Alexander 1992; Schaffer 1992; Frazer & Sechrist 1994; Cushway 1995). If such studies are to be used effectively there needs to be a selective and informed approach from the wide range available to give credence to a specific argument.

Research into staff support can offer supportive evidence when making a case for resources or a staff support system. As yet there are few standard or nationally used criteria to go by, so comparisons and generalisations can only be made with some caution if integrity is to be maintained. Research may be *qualitative or quantitative* but does not necessarily fit into these categories, partly due to the range of variables involved. Moss (1995) points out that *action research* may offer a more practical approach for looking at staff support. This includes a range of strategies using an *interpretative approach*, involving staff in the process and involving them in planning action needed. There is an element in this kind of study of the Hawthorne effect (Hawthorne 1932) which describes how, when a group knows it is being observed, there is improved performance and group morale. Any data collected will reflect any effects of the changes introduced, so it is important that the changes are measurable. The process itself is important in action research as it also helps to keep the group members informed and knowledgeable about the subject, allowing them to contribute creative ideas. Staff co-operate more readily with any action introduced if it results from research to which they have contributed.

Serious research can be time consuming and costly if it is to be effective and its validity acceptable. Information of some kind is often required in a very short time to support a proposal. Here the audit process and monitoring can be useful in producing some immediate results indicating good and bad practices relating to staff support, effectiveness and morale.

Monitoring and auditing

Monitoring is an ongoing process linked to research. Monitoring and audit are simple tools used to judge the various aspects of organisational life or to evaluate a small sample of the total population. They are important in the current internal market where purchasers have to be convinced by providers that they deliver services at the level agreed. This is applicable to staff support as, if staff are not well managed and supported, there is a detrimental effect on all aspects of the organisation's life. The use of monitoring and audit (including personal appraisal or individual reviews) should help to identify *training needs* of individuals and groups of staff and shortfalls in skills provision which need to be addressed. It also gives an overall picture of the effectiveness of the organisation and the efficiency of selection criteria. It should help to form job descriptions and personal specifications for each job and to focus attention on requirements for further education and training.

Monitoring and audit are very similar. *Monitoring* is an ongoing regulatory process looking at individuals, teams and the organisation and is a natural part of the management process to keep an eye on what is happening. *Audit* can be described more as a 'snapshot approach', taking a look at how a group or the organisation is performing as seen from the outside, using the evidence of the monitoring processes and specific audit tools to evaluate progress achieved against objectives. There are many monitoring tools already in use that can be part of the specific audit procedure, such as records of sickness and absenteeism, the kind of complaints made by staff or patients, staff morale, or changes in the quality of care. The audit process requires the setting of objectives applicable to the particular organisation and the particular team. This process can help to identify good and bad issues relating to staff support.

An important point to note is that the absence of staff care and support is often more immediately obvious than its presence, which mirrors attitudes relating to health, i.e. people become aware of their health when they are ill. Good staff support is evidenced by good team work, good team communication, courtesy to one another and awareness of one another, including issues relating to life outside work, such as family and social life. It is also evident through improved individual and team morale, high performance levels, low sickness and absence rates and a creative and pleasant atmosphere.

Audit processes address all aspects of the organisation and it is important to assess outcomes and not just the process. Needs, expectations and goals also need clarification. Audit is a well recognised management tool and quite applicable to staff support, as outcomes aid the individual staff member and also the quality of the team and of patient care (Farman & Gore 1995).

Presenting an action plan for staff support

A well argued case for staff support will need to start by stating the philosophy of that particular organisation, and the agreed definition and mission statement which will be a clear indication of the parameters within which the presentation is made. It is useful to have a well thought out strategic plan for selecting and presenting evidence, and preparing a plan for action. There are four main stages to consider:

(1) Assessing the resources available
(2) Selecting and collating the evidence, including identification of local needs, and evidence from those who have a system in place
(3) Preparing a plan of action
(4) Formulating a well documented proposal for a staff support system.

Assessing the resources

The check list in Table 9.1 is a useful guide and once completed will offer an opportunity to bring together a group of identified staff who are both interested and supportive. It will assist those who already have skills in staff support or are involved in some kind of supportive service and are interested in developing it further. By being involved in the participitative process, staff are more likely to 'own' and to support the agreed course of action.

A vital contribution will be to *identify* the resources available locally, as in Table 9.1. It will then be important to identify the areas of greatest need and the problems specific to the organisation. There will be areas where it is known that pressures generally run high or there are occasions of sudden severe traumatic incidents e.g. intensive care unit, accident and emergency department or paediatrics. Less obvious are areas where sickness/absenteeism figures are unexpectedly high if compared with the average, or where there is discontent because of unsatisfactory relationships or feelings of being unfairly treated. Such areas will need to be given priority. Other assessments mentioned elsewhere in this text could be used to highlight local pressures or weaknesses that need attention, perhaps in the selection of staff or role

Table 9.1 Assessing existing resources for support systems (Channon *et al.*, 1992).

It will help identify your needs if you assess first your present resources. Fill in a few comments on each of the areas outlined below, and identify a contact person in each field.

Resources	**Contact person**
(1) Existing services	
(a) Counselling	
(b) Occupational health service	
(c) Chaplaincy department	
(d) Other, e.g. external provision, psychologist, etc.	
(2) Educational facilities*	
(a) In basic courses – medicine, nursing etc.	
(b) In-service training or post basic courses	
(c) Specific short courses, e.g. self awareness or development	
(d) Provision for specialist training, e.g. counselling course.	
(3) Financial resources	
(a) Allocation for posts	
(b) Allocation for resources, e.g. training, travel, etc.	
(c) Replacement staff for time out relief, sickness etc.	
(4) Key individuals	
(a) Name some staff members who could be approached in developing support services, e.g. unit manager, psychology lecturer, etc.	
(b) Name some staff members who might have some suitable skills already, or who show potential for this kind of support, and given some encouragement and training would be key persons in a crucial area, e.g. a unit manager in an intensive care department.	

* Financial resources already allocated should be included here.

allocation. It is likely that members of the planning group will be able to give some indication where the most vulnerable spots are, and then various tools could be used to verify this, or the extent of the pressures or causes etc. Presentation of local needs to indicate priorities is a vital part of the evidence.

Selecting and collating evidence

Ideally evidence in support of the proposal should come from two different sources:

(1) Evidence of needs, priorities and resources available in that particular organisation
(2) Evidence selected from national research findings on the cost and effects of untreated stress and the benefits of good staff support.

Evidence on costs and benefits to the organisation

When a proposal is being prepared for setting up a staff support system, one of the first questions asked will be, 'What is it going to cost – can we afford it?'. There are no simple answers, except perhaps to say, 'Can you afford to be without it?'. Resource committees will be looking for hard facts to convince them that the proposition is worthwhile. The difficulty is that hard facts are not readily available in relation to this topic, partly because it is not the easiest topic to research and on which to present figures which are universal or will convince. However, good use can be made of the *existing information* to present a strong supporting argument specifically suitable for a particular organisation, and one which will be convincing to the managers.

The evidence relating to *local needs* can be compiled using some of the assessment tools suggested in Chapters 3 and 6. In the short term the local information available may be incomplete but can be augmented from existing monitoring and audit systems. Statistics on absenteeism and sickness are an example of information that organisations will have available. This information is necessary for organisations to plan staffing levels, as sickness costs affect managers' budgets. Care is necessary in measuring absence rates as accuracy can be affected by the presence of part-time staff, methods of calculating working days, or the effects of shift systems. Helpful suggestions for accurate calculations can be found in a practical guide (Health at Work in the NHS 1995b).

Another phenomenon, described by Cooper *et al.* (1996), is that of 'presenteeism'. This describes the situation where staff remain at work when they are unwell, and so are a possible risk to patient care and are vulnerable themselves. Staff may do this because of a fear of losing the job or jeopardising promotion prospects. The effects may include mistakes in drug administration, failure to pass on essential information or increased accident risks.

In the context of *work related stress* the element of *risk* is an important one often overlooked. Staff can be a risk to themselves or patients because of excessive pressures in the work load, or their personal response to pressures, or ill health and exhaustion. Risk can also be caused by hazards in the working environment, or inadequate supervision, or lack of resources and equipment (Griffiths *et al.* 1996).

Other costs to the organisation will be evident in areas like time keeping, accident rates, decision making, staff relationships and aggravation, and poor industrial relations, to quote a few (Cox *et al.* 1990). Cox suggests the health of an organisation has a 'Gestalt quality – being more than the sum of its parts', that is more than the sum of the health of individuals.

Selecting evidence from other sources

Any resourcing committee will want a good reason for allocating scarce resources to staff support. They will be looking for evidence on three aspects:

(1)   The costs to the organisation of *failing to provide* staff support services
(2)   The *costs of providing* a support system and what it entails
(3)   The *benefits* that will accrue from having a staff support policy.

They will need to be persuaded by a reasoned and logical argument that:

(1)   Failure to consider this issue is *costly*, to the organisation and individual
(2)   They can *maximise the use of resources* by considering a plan to meet their particular local needs
(3)   There will be *tangible benefits* to the organisation and individual as a result of their action and policy.

Careful selection of the most appropriate evidence available, which is relevant to the local situation, can make a powerful case. Selection can be bewildering for those surveying the range of different approaches but there is guidance available. Many of the references quoted in this book will offer useful material, and selection can be made looking at costs and benefits to:

(1) The individual
(2) The team
(3) The organisation.

This will ensure a comprehensive approach and is likely to lead to a balanced outcome and enhanced benefits. It is helpful to use quoted evidence to develop the argument in a logical sequence. There are the well known *costs to the individual* in terms of stress related illness and lowered efficiency and here Cooper's studies provide good documentation (Cooper 1988; Cooper *et al.* 1996). Long before the cumulative effects of pressure manifest themselves in more serious illness, the individual's quality of life can be diminished, which can be translated into poor performance at work, general irritability and lowered immunity (Cox 1993). The effects eventually hit the *team* and the *organisation* in terms of low performance and increased absenteeism, both of which contribute to increasing costs. The human side of this in terms of individual unhappiness is often overlooked in the attempt to consider the financial implications.

Taking a wider view, it is important to reflect that untreated pressures also affect the *costs* to the *National Health Service* and to *the nation as a whole*. The media constantly bombard the public with figures relating to the nation's health and the effects of stress related illnesses, showing that results are often higher for staff in health care services. A figure for short term absence, 25% of which may well be influenced by workplace pressures, is quoted in NASS (1992a). The Royal College of Nursing estimated in 1991 that savings of about £6.4 million could be made by reducing the annual nurse wastage rate from 25% to 15% annually, and there is a strong correlation between pressures and attrition (Birch 1975).

An example of a logical way of selecting and using relevant material on costs and benefits can be seen in a paper published by NASS (1992a). It is important to present material which relates to the particular proposal in hand, and to use it to support the argument. For example, there is clear evidence that certain health care professional groups have higher mortality and morbidity rates than the general population. A report by the BMA (1993) quotes detailed evidence on occupational morbidity and mortality for doctors. Compared with other professionals, doctors are more likely to have poor marriage relationships, greater use of sleeping pills or drugs to help them to cope, and more alcohol problems. They have a 72% greater risk of suicide than the population as a whole.

Statistical evidence is often more readily available for businesses and organisations in industry, where greater significance is attached to the welfare of the workforce. Cox (1993) gives a comprehensive summary of the research evidence that can be used to highlight vulnerable groups and potentially damaging situations in the workplace.

Benefits of staff support and stress management

There are two kinds of costs which have to be considered and balanced against each other, when making an evaluation of the *benefits* of stress management. The costs of providing staff support services must be set against the costs which will accrue if the situation is ignored, and these days that could be very expensive with litigation becoming evident, not just for physical results of neglect but also psychological.

Research in this area is not yet plentiful as it takes time to implement schemes and demonstrate benefits. A report on costs and benefits to organisations (Cooper *et al.* 1996) gives information on three case studies in Europe on *stress prevention in the workplace*. It offers general information on the costs of workplace stress, which is useful for supportive evidence. For example:

- Staff have the biggest impact on costs for an organisation, accounting for 50–80% of expenditure
- 40% of respondents considered work activity affected health and 42% of these referred to stress
- Total costs of work related sickness account for between 2.5% and 10.1% when expressed as a percentage of gross national product (GNP)
- In the UK 360 million working days are lost each year through sickness, at a cost to organisations of £8 billion; at least half of these are related to workplace stress
- The overall cost of occupational stress in the UK amounts to over 10% of GNP.

As the UK National Health Service is one of the largest employers in Europe, it is easy to see how significant such figures are.

The three case studies recorded in the report of Cooper *et al.* (1996) are valuable assessments of different approaches in industry, from which lessons can be learned. The conclusions reached show that:

- Organisations tend to introduce secondary and tertiary level prevention (concerned with stress awareness and stress management skills)

- Primary prevention is more frequently overlooked (which relates to reducing the stressors)
- Secondary and tertiary levels as 'stand alone initiatives' are not the complete answer unless addressed simultaneously with eliminating the sources of stress.

These findings, together with Cartwright's work (Cartwright 1996) discussed in Chapter 5, can give a sense of direction when formulating a proposal.

A study of mental health among NHS staff (Borrill *et al.* 1996), which was commissioned by the Department of Health and carried out at Sheffield University, reported some important findings which can be used in supporting a proposal:

- 26.8% of staff in NHS trusts experience poor mental health
- There are differences across occupational groups – among managers 33.4% were identified as probable cases of psychiatric disorder, compared with 28.5% of nurses and 27.8% of doctors
- The mental health of staff in the NHS is substantially poorer than those working outside the NHS
- Female employees tend to show significantly higher figures than males, and a number of work related factors are associated with these differences
- The mental health of staff differs between trusts.

One finding Moore (1996) elaborates on is that the differences between trusts indicated that staff in trusts where 'there was greater co-operation, better communications and more freedom for staff decision making' showed mental health ratings *twice as good* as the other trusts.

Tangible benefits such as this are still in a minority as studies of the value of interventions are still few, but those that have been completed are encouraging and positive (Cooper *et al.* 1996). A survey of employee assistance programmes in 1991 (IRS 1991) reported that benefits to employers included:

- Reports on improved individual performance
- Reductions in absenteeism
- Improved employee relationships
- Preventive aspects such as a drop in alcoholism
- Improved morale and general feelings among staff of being cared for
- Reduced accident rates and insurance costs.

Some other sources of information on benefits can be found in NASS (1992a).

One other potential cost/benefit is the growing awareness that organisations can incur enormous costs if damages are awarded following litigation, as seen in the *Walker* case (*Walker* v. *Northumberland County Council* 1994 IRLR 35). John Walker won £170,000 as a result of his claims for damages due to pressures from his workload (Jones 1995). The Royal College of Nursing points out that it can only be a matter of time before there are cases to be heard from nurses and others (Moore 1996). Proper staff support systems and policies can protect against such potential damaging costs.

The few examples quoted here indicate that there is material from which to select (NASS 1992a), and show how this can be used to support a proposal to good advantage. It is possible to indicate what the possible benefits of a proposal are, and although these are not easy to demonstrate, a strong argument can be given to support the discussion (Hingley & Marks 1991).

Preparing an action plan

The content of the action plan will be governed by the nature of the factual material obtained and will include:

- Assessment of needs relating to the work situation and the nature of the job
- Agreement on priorities
- Resources already in place which can be enhanced, extended or developed
- New resources which are known to be available
- The overall organisational culture – attitudes of employees and management
- Opportunity and facilities for staff in-service training and resources for this
- Communication channels and their effectiveness
- Facilities for staff support services and access for all staff
- Choice of the appropriate services to be established to meet the organisation's need
- Choice of monitoring/evaluation and review services.

In addition to these considerations the process of decision making in formulating this plan is vital to its success. It needs:

- To be *'owned' and affirmed* by management following the considerations described above
- To be *'owned' by individuals* throughout the organisation at all levels
- To be acceptable to all participants as being a right and proper way of receiving and giving care and support
- To reflect the managerial structure and philosophy.

A system should be built into the plan for regular monitoring, updating and review.

Formulating and presenting a proposal

Formulating a proposal is an important aspect of the whole process and should reflect the research evidence and consultation that has been part of the preparation. The nature of the presentation will be influenced by the kind of body to receive it – what their attitudes, priorities and preferences are likely to be, and the element of competition from other deserving causes within the organisation. Careful consideration is needed of the appropriate issues and how to select and present priorities.

Ideally the presentation should give collated evidence to support a logical argument for the strategic plan that is being put forward. It needs to embrace the main areas described in this chapter, and will include the organisation's agreed philosophy of staff support and mission statement. The presentation needs to be concise and to the point; committee members have many papers to digest and are more likely to pay full attention to two or three pages clearly set out than to ten pages of detailed material. Points to be addressed could include:

- Philosophy of staff support
- A general statement on the need for staff support based on costs and benefits and examples selected from national figures
- The process of consultation and methods of assessment used locally
- Names and roles of employees participating in the planning group
- A report on causes and origins of pressures, identifying 'hot spots', needs and priorities in the organisation
- Identification of existing resources/services which are already available and could be enhanced or expanded

- Outline of resources needed to maximise the support offered or suggestions of how they could be redistributed.

This should be followed by an action plan identifying priorities and presenting a strategic outline for short, medium and long term development together with built-in evaluation and review procedures.

Such a proposal embraces the needs of the whole organisation. It is likely to succeed if there is ongoing participation from employees at all levels, and if a definitive plan is accepted it may need to be modified from time to time in the light of resources available.

As shown by research findings, a comprehensive and integrated approach involving the workforce, rather than being imposed by management, is likely to produce real benefits. Some of the key issues to be considered, however, are easily overlooked as they are less tangible. These will include ensuring *good consultation procedures*, *participation* of the workforce which brings a sense of *ownership*, with staff feeling *valued*, and above all a willingness to change the *culture* where necessary. Finally the whole process needs constant *reappraisal* to ensure *flexibility* and *adaptation* in response to need in a constantly changing culture.

Key points

(1) Research, monitoring and audit are all useful approaches to assessing staff support needs.
(2) Making a case for a staff support system involves participation and discussion at all levels.
(3) The process involves assessment of needs and resources, selecting supportive evidence, preparing an action plan and formulating and presenting a proposal.
(4) The costs and benefits presented can be drawn from both national and local resources.
(5) A supportive culture is essential to the success of any policy adopted.

Exercises

(9.1) Consider the nature of monitoring, audit and research, and give an example of how one of these tools could be used for an investigation in staff support in your workplace.

(9.2) Identify and outline some of the support services available in your organisation. How could these be used more effectively?

(9.3) Consider the supportive culture and ethos of care in your organisation. How would you suggest this could be improved?

Section IV

The Workplace in the Wider World Context

Chapter 10

Current Realities – Philosophies and Specifics

'And now that we know the principle, we can look at its applications. As we have likely recognised by now, no two snowflakes, trees or animals are alike. No two people are the same, either. Everything has its own inner nature.'

Benjamin Hoff: *The Tao of Pooh*

Formulating a policy

Formulating a policy involves considering a range of principles and is more than just writing down a simple statement. The ultimate statement may be short and to the point, but it can only be relevant if consideration has been given to the current facts, needs and values of the particular organisation, and this must be apparent in any accompanying document. Some of the practical aspects of preparing a policy for staff support were mentioned briefly in Chapter 6. This section develops the subject within the context of building on particular philosophies.

The health care services, whether voluntary or statutory, are ultimately about providing good quality care for those in need. Any organisation that cares for its staff is likely to be successful in all aspects of its provision of care. All good and really successful organisations care for their staff. Sometimes this is apparent in recruitment advertising and is an important selling point when seeking new staff with similar values.

While carers may respond to the need to care for themselves, they may limit their approach to ideas expressed in jargon such as 'I need some space', which is one way in which people indicate a need but avoid exploring the real needs. This particular jargon may really be just a plea for someone to say 'thank you'. A clearly stated policy will avoid some of the misunderstandings that may occur.

This emphasises the need for a clear policy statement on care, even if it states the obvious like offering dignity and respect to the individual, and it should express the beliefs of an organisation and spell out their importance in terms of delivery of staff care.

Any good organisation will recognise that staff support is an important ingredient for success. This recognition is desirable at all levels and needs to be apparent in any mission statement of that organisation. It must be seen to be practised by senior managers, within teams, by unit managers or by leaders in education, including each member of staff, and support needs to be evident between colleagues and team members. Each individual is encouraged to recognise and respect personal needs for support, proper recreation and management of lifestyle.

For any carer to care adequately for others it is essential for:

- The carer to feel cared for
- The carer to be and to feel valued
- Each member of a team to care for themselves and each other if the team is to be effective and function well
- The organisation and members of the team to care for each member and value their role, to enable optimum performance
- Management to care about the delivery of the caring function and the members who hold the responsibility of that function, encouraging care at each level.

This underlying principle of care is inherent in the nature of the service the organisation has to deliver and it is impossible to formulate a good policy if there is no underlying acceptance of the philosophy of care. This preferably needs to have emerged over a period of years and to be part of the culture of the organisation.

A good example of this can be seen in the trend to provide charters of various kinds for the care of the customer, consumer or patient. They give a statement of policy and the preparation does involve thinking through the fundamental aspects of the service, and in some way setting a standard for expectations. They may appear to state the obvious but they do provide an opportunity to express values and beliefs about standards. In health care this includes points like waiting times, postponement of surgery, etc. Charters are a record of what is important to a policy of care, as they

(Contd)

record what is uncaring and detrimental to reaching standards set. They indicate what standards are desirable and draw attention to something that requires action. In this way charters help towards making a policy statement.

A decision to adopt a staff support charter is an important first step towards action as it does at least show that there is a policy for staff support. Some trusts and health authorities have prepared charters for staff support to suit their own needs. A policy which has been adopted by a number of trusts was prepared by a group of experts in staff support provision from a range of organisations and was co-ordinated and published in 1992 by NASS as a Charter for Staff Support in Health Care. A policy may include consideration of practical staff care, such as provision for proper meal times, relaxation, time-out. It may include opportunities for staff to request further training for specific roles, for facilities for career guidance, and for information on resources available. Such a policy may be written up in the form of a charter.

A particular team may wish to formulate its own policy to address their speciality, or a single or multidisciplinary policy may be appropriate. A policy needs to show care for staff at all levels of the organisation. It looks at the aims and sets up values, then the means, for achieving these. Policies also affect and reflect the public image of the organisation in the outside world. A powerful first impression is created in the process of appointing new staff. A proper information pack is essential, incliuding accurate directions, and on arrival it is important to be welcomed and to be looked after both before and after the interview. Opportunity should be given for feedback to unsuccessful candidates. This all depicts the ability of an organisation to care for its staff and establishes some important principles about care being an integral part of the system.

From principles to practice

The principles discussed here can be used with the practical points set out at the beginning of Chapter 6, as the foundation for a policy designed specifically for a particular organisation. We have already noted the importance of recognising the cultural setting in which the staff find themselves (Chapter 6) and this involves recognition of current trends. At the time of writing we are living in a world of constant change. The expectations of security of a job for life or of permanent employment in a particular career are difficult to sustain. Even the nature of the job may change. The most important part of a job description to be aware of is the open-ended part with phrases like 'other duties as required'. This puts particular pressure on those who find change and adaptation difficult.

In today's work situation the dominant attitude required is adaptability: the need to adapt to change within the job, changes within the organisation and the changing needs of society at large.

> 'We trained very hard, but it seemed that every time we were beginning to form up into teams, we would be reorganised. I was to learn later in life that we tend to meet every situation by reorganising and a wonderful method it can be for creating the illusion of progress, while producing confusion, inefficiency and demoralisation.'

> Gaius Petronius (AD 66)

One of the greatest stressors, particularly for those who only feel safe operating within set parameters, is that they may have the same title as someone else but be carrying out a completely different job. This is so for all professions both inside and outside the health service. Each job evolves, and like all other aspects of evolution you either adapt or you become 'extinct' (Toffler 1971).

Sea based creatures can go through an evolutionary process until they become land based, which means they have to grow lungs. In other words, if they don't adapt they become extinct.

Toffler suggested that the best way to adapt was to have a number of options prepared in readiness for potential changes, and these could be put into practice at the opportune moment. Individuals prepared in this way will be the survivors. He also stresses the importance of being able to tackle new ventures in 'small bite-sized pieces'. This way innovators are less likely to be discouraged and so will avoid the stress of failure.

Being 'extinct' in terms of jobs means that the job 'dies' so the person has to go, or the employment ends because the person sees they cannot cope or someone else sees this for them. This can be linked to lack of job satisfaction, or early retirement or retirement on the grounds of ill health. When a person does not adapt to changes they will increasingly feel like a square peg in a round hole and will be out of focus with the organisation and the team. No longer are the needs of the job and the aims of the individual matched.

Increasingly one criterion for jobs in caring professions needs to be the capacity to adapt. People can be divided roughly into two groups. One group sees change as threatening, destructive or even retrograde. They look back to a golden age when everything was supposedly as it should be. The other group know the past was not so golden at the time, and they accept the challenge of change and are energised to respond to it.

> In a study from the Royal College of Nursing Research Unit a number of community nurses were reported as saying they would much prefer to go back to the old style of 'nursing superintendent or matron' than to work under the current style of manager. In fact most of these community nurses were not old enough to have worked under the old regime or they might have thought differently (Traynor & Wade 1992).

Among the first group mentioned above, a resistance to or blocking of change can be evident, which is an attempt to hold the situation or turn the clock back. This puts people into a situation of conflict, whereas those who see change as an opportunity for the development of the service, the development of care, or self development, view it as a challenge. Change needs managing and it needs action. It needs to be analysed quickly, to be understood and to be responded to in a creative way. This leads to job satisfaction at a high level for those who do change, because to be innovative and part of an innovative venture, and to know one is responding, is to know that one is doing something creative, which is highly satisfying.

In order to do this the person needs to feel safe to experiment, safe to try and to risk making mistakes, feeling supported and valued throughout. Innovation always demands high levels of team work where each team member is able to participate in sharing ideas, but also has additional roles in experimenting and developing those ideas, so limiting mistakes and misunderstandings and potential damage. Each member can also play a part in evaluating results and feeding new knowledge into practice, or creating new areas of research.

This creative response to change means each member of the team has a responsibility to share in the development of new ways to meet present and future situations. Senior managers are not the only ones to participate in creative ideas; they can harness the valuable resource available to them throughout the organisation.

Current realities in the work place

Staff support needs tuning to the demands and pressures of each particular area and team, also to the individual members within those teams. So responses need to be adaptable to a range of different situations.

The broad principles of staff support are universal, but their application is specific to particular areas of need. Response takes account of all needs but then identifies particular problems and pressures, and the unique demands of that particular area. Responses which will be helpful are identified.

The support services offered need to take into account:

- Universal needs of all staff
- Specific needs of particular groups which may need local consideration, and on particular occasions emergency provision as required
- Cultivation of an overall caring culture
- Need for services provided to be known and accessible to all staff.

Universal needs include the basic needs of all staff in health care as already identified in Section III of this book, and include personal and work based needs. Provisions need to be in place and accessible for all staff at all times. Examples include proper provision of health care, occupational health, health and safety policies, counselling support, training and education. An example of a need which can arise occasionally is when a bereavement occurs; support and understanding should be available at all such times.

To some extent all situations have special dimensions, but some are more acute and damaging than others if neglected, so as well as defining the nature of the universal provision of support, it is important to consider the *specific needs* of each team, department, speciality or organisation. Specific needs are not confined to emergency areas of service but can be ongoing and can occur when the nature of the work is repetitive, boring or exhausting. The work may require constant high standards of demanding care, such as in caring for elderly people or those with limited mobility or facilities. Special support is needed on a regular basis, as it is in areas like paediatrics, intensive care or any area involving fast changing technology and quick adaptation to change.

Application of research experience may be valuable here. For example, studies show that junior doctors or nursing staff are more regularly exposed to trauma in the ward and have less experience to deal with it than the consultant or ward sister. This needs recognition and special provision made for that group, maybe in the form of special debriefing.

Unexpected incidents always present a dramatic scenario, where good anticipation and preparation for any emergency are essential because no one knows when or how disaster will strike or which units will receive the impact. This is a specific area requiring both built-in provision and immediate response to the unknown. If good support is not available post traumatic stress disorder may be a long term sequel.

Specific groups, such as some professional groups, may have continuous particular support needs, for example staff in the area of mental health, particularly dealing with ethical and attitude problems. This is expanded in the next chapter. Community care staff have different kinds of pressures needing support. For example, they might be isolated from colleagues or might experience professional differences within a general practice unit. Then there are emergency services such as ambulance staff who face both ongoing or particular crises at different times, or staff working in HIV/AIDS who again have very special needs for support.

Another need may arise for staff dealing with a situation in different professions or at different levels of responsibility or with different roles. For example, the consultant may be ultimately responsible for a decision to terminate life support but it may fall to more junior staff to carry the pressures of actually turning off the machine and dealing with the distraught relatives. Some of the pressure arises when staff are appointed to posts where they do not have the ability or experience to handle the situations which confront them, or to adapt to the pressures. This again emphasises the importance of good selection procedures and in-service training as part of the wider spectrum of staff support.

Other dimensions

We have considered universal needs, specific support care, ongoing support care and care for particular groups. All these need recognition and provision in preparing a staff support policy.

Preparing a policy involves consideration of selecting and appointing staff, in-service training and development, attitudes to oneself and others, valuing oneself and others, and seeing how this is costed out in the individual's situation. For example, it means making sure that management of staff support is applied to a specific area; that communications are effective and can be understood; and that training programmes are identified to build up the regular skills and attitudes appropriate to that particular area. There needs to be a range of places to which people can go across the institution, where training needs can be met and which will include group work specific to a particular area. For example, debriefing procedures would need to be a much stronger element in intensive care or accident and emergency than they would in caring for the elderly or working in the community. In the latter it may be more necessary to focus attention on the cumulative effects of pressures arising from isolation or dealing with chronic illness, or feelings of being undervalued and part of a 'Cinderella' service.

There are other situations, for example where a manager is constantly introducing change for change's sake. Little consideration is given to past records or the possibility of success, or to the disruption it can cause perhaps with little achievement other than creating high levels of tension for staff and affecting the whole team morale. Such a person may be needing to stamp their own authority or create an impression of activity to enhance their own power base by making everyone else feel insecure. This may take the form of constantly moving staff around between posts, or of changing areas of responsibility or of introducing new structures without reference to those who have to implement them. This maverick attitude to change is not uncommon and can create high stress levels all round, with consequent effects on performance as the goal posts are frequently moved and there are no points of reference – either from previous situations or from information during the period of change – to provide some pattern to work to and reset the goals.

Other areas which are part of the fabric of the organisation and need attention are:

(1) The need to give good education and ongoing in-service training to help build the highest level of professional knowledge. Where up-to-date information is available this may be brought to bear on decision making and this can reduce the conflict levels and stresses of feeling inadequate to make judgements.

(2) It is important to draw together the multidisciplinary team who are involved with difficult situations. This gives a more realistic

understanding of what each agency can achieve and treatment is enhanced by co-operation.
(3) Support needs to be given to those involved at the sharp end of the service to help them handle difficult interactions with patients and families, for example handling anger, aggression and violence, verbal and physical.

Example of specific provision for staff support

Response to disaster situations

This chapter has focused on the importance of stating a basic philosophy and formulating a policy which is practical and will lead to efficient functioning in real situations. This often involves specific plans to meet particular needs. Major disasters attract much attention, including media, public and professional interest in post traumatic stress disorder (PTSD). This is used here to illustrate how support needs in a specific situation can be approached, as the principles used can readily be adapted for many other special areas of need.

It is clearly a situation requiring immediate response from staff and involving a very obvious requirement for staff support. Also, a major incident involves a complexity of services ranging through community, emergency hospitals and voluntary services. It also includes the often unrecognised aspect of the *personal* effects of disaster which can be equally traumatic and can have a wide ranging impact on family relationships, for onlookers at the scene or those carrying on other regular duties for the emergency staff (Rose 1995). Because major disasters are now widely recognised as leading to post traumatic stress disorder, if untreated, (Meekin 1990; Rose 1994; Rosser 1994), this is a good example of how support for needs in special areas can be approached.

The process involves identification of needs and the course of action required, including recognition of the following:

• The immediate needs at the site of disaster
• Support for individuals at the site – staff, victims and onlookers
• Support in the receiving units – A and E, theatre, intensive care, etc.
• Support in dealing with the uncertainty of unknown situations
• The needs of families and relatives
• Involvement of other services

- Involving outside help for staff support
- Long term provision for after effects.

One aspect which should be recognised is the need to differentiate between a 'designated major disaster' and a 'personal' or 'little' disaster, as the same principles apply in each case. The personal disasters are easily overlooked but they can occur at any time and as a result of cumulative pressures which, if unrecognised and untreated, lead to a state of imbalance and build up over time until there is a 'trigger' which pushes the individual into a state of PTSD (Stoter 1995b).

Preparation involves aspects which may well already be in place and an ongoing provision, but will need to be focused directly on to this issue, including:

- Identification of specific needs of various groups involved
- Responding to those needs, long and short term
- Training for aspects of response
- Regular updating through education
- Establishing the value and practice of good team work
- Ensuring support networks are in place and functioning
- Ensuring professionals feel safe, competent and confident in clearly defined roles
- Ensuring they understand each other's roles
- Incorporating these points in well thought out plans.

Every major disaster has its own features, and how, when or where a major incident will happen is clearly unpredictable. This in itself means that preparation must be good so that staff can be confident of a good structure behind them, and can feel that they know and can depend on their colleagues throughout the service. The centre of control needs to be clearly identified for each aspect of provision. Knowing where reserve services can be found is also important, to avoid overloading staff especially where critical skills are necessary, for example in the operating theatre or for decision making.

Other needs for staff will include:

- Careful selection and identification of those leading various areas
- Rest and refreshment facilities
- Access to immediate debriefing services
- Longer term counselling where necessary
- Arrangement for 'time out' when individual members have had enough pressure.

It is important to work out a specific plan in the local context, as it brings together the local leaders of services to plan and work through a local strategy, identify resources and agree how to co-ordinate operational services. This process ensures that they have had face to face contact and have learned to value and respect one another and understand each other's strengths and limitations of resources, thus helping to establish teamwork and avoid 'competition'. The principle ingredients of each plan will include and build on those outlined in Section I of this book and will draw further on more recent literature, research and experience, including the following key points:

- A *well structured plan* identifying all key persons involved.
- Clarification of *areas of responsibility*, and circulation of this information to staff in all local services.
- *Good communication systems* between all services and departments.
- *Arrangements to provide a shift system* to maintain high standards around the clock by providing respite to carers. This applies to all disciplines and agencies.
- A regular programme of *in-service education*, to develop awareness of need, recognition of signs of distress and acceptance of the value of support, with regular refresher training to retain confidence.
- Adequate *debriefing arrangements*, both on the spot and formalised ones later within disciplines and also multidisciplinary.
- Arrangements for '*dry run*' rehearsals and regular reappraisal of plans.
- Maintaining a *caring culture* for staff at all times.
- Having a well-established support system in place.
- *Readiness to learn* from all experiences and modify plans in the light of evidence.

This plan can be used as a model for staff support planning in many special areas as the same basic philosophy of care, policy and planning is involved in each case.

There is a wider and more complex dimension involving staff support, which is increasingly a matter of concern. It concerns those dealing with difficult ethical situations, embracing painful choices and conflicting values. There are worries for managers and organisations with the growing possibility of legal liability, and this is a significant motivator for staff support provision. This leads into the wider arena of difficult issues requiring specific support, which are the subject of the next chapter.

The principles underlying the formation of any plan involving major disaster are basic and general, although every organisation will find it useful to anticipate various scenarios, in order to evaluate the responses available and their accessibility. It may not be obvious at first that this is related to staff support, but all the procedures ensure that the preventive aspects are included, damaging effects are limited and support is built in as required.

The *regular re-appraisal of plans and modification* in the light of new experience is essential, as is the provision for a 'dry run' at intervals to ensure the efficient co-ordination of services. By their nature disasters are sudden, unexpected and unpredictable, but the disruption and trauma of such unpredictability can be kept to a minimum given the presence of good planning and team co-operation, with staff trained to respond and adapt to the challenge, in both the short and long term.

This kind of approach presents an excellent example of 'rethinking' between professionals and across boundaries. It ensures the sharing of and best use of skills, the establishment of good communications, and an approach that limits the damaging effects of trauma and makes provision for ongoing staff care. It serves as an example of how principles can be applied both within and between organisations.

Key points

(1) Formulating a policy on staff support involves a range of principles and the identification of specific needs.

(2) The principles agreed need to be the basis for a practical working document.

(3) The policy needs to be flexible enough to change with changing situations, and to have the capacity to adapt to changing needs.

(4) Provision needs to be made for universal and specific needs, and to prepare for unexpected demands.

(5) One example is given of preparing a specific policy relating to major disasters.

Exercises

(10.1) Think about the principles you would use in formulating a staff support policy in your particular workplace. Outline the philosophy of care you would suggest as a basis for your policy. Identify any specific needs to be considered and set out the priorities in terms of principles, and the priorities of the needs identified.

(10.2) How would you propose to make your policy work effectively?

(10.3) Make a list of the people in your organisation who could be involved in a planning group considering preparation for disaster. Discuss the value of having such a group participating in the planning together.

Chapter 11

Attitudes and Values – Mix and Match

Attitudes and values are assuming growing importance where the need for staff support is concerned. They can give rise to conflicts in a number of difficult areas, each bringing their own pressures and highlighting many complex issues. This means staff support needs to be given careful consideration and thought for those working in *specialist* areas.

Values are basic foundations for social life and influence the way people live and behave. They are related to attitudes and beliefs and affect how we make decisions and resolve conflicts. Beliefs are often related to faith rather than fact. Values may change but beliefs tend to be more permanent (Tschudin 1992). Ethics are also involved with ways of behaving, concerned with responsibility in society and therefore related to many matters of concern to health care workers.

Areas of conflict

The caring professions, particularly those more immediately involved with health, were founded on a tradition of care and of service given to those in need. The majority of staff in these occupations are there because they want to give a service of good quality care. Today values tend to focus more on business and management principles; people are more preoccupied with resource management, budgeting and efficiency. This can give rise to conflict leading to severe pressures. Whereas in business the notion of profit is to the fore, it is difficult in health care to provide an adequate and efficient service let alone enter into a profit making arena. Resources are limited and budgets have to balance, purchasers and providers feature prominently, and health care staff often feel the patients' interests and needs are relegated to second place and it is difficult to sustain a caring ethos. Pressure arising from conflicts of this nature can be painful and exhausting.

Rights and responsibilities

Ethical considerations involve rights and responsibilities. Rights are concerned with human needs and are often overemphasised to the exclusion of responsibilities, and we fail to notice that rights and responsibilities go together. Responsibilities are rarely mentioned with rights, while rights are frequently a topic of interest to journalists and others. This area can be a source of conflict between employers, managers and staff when the responsibility aspects are overlooked and rights and responsibilities clearly belong together for each group.

Other general areas relating to attitudes, prejudices and conflict include ethical and racial issues which may give rise to staff feeling undervalued. There may be evidence of discrimination, giving rise to conflicting values and difficulties in relationships. Such pressures also relate to bullying, harassment and violence, all of which may lead to conflicts, and staff involved will need special support to meet these situations, as well as policies being built in to prevent such things having a detrimental and cumulative effect.

Special difficulties

Staff in special areas can feel themselves to be different, and that conflicts relating to basic needs do not apply to them. Specialist areas such as intensive care units and accident and emergency departments can develop a specific culture and sometimes it appears as a rather black sense of humour. There can be an identity which is about uniqueness and conformity within the group, bringing an internal sense of solidarity for the group. For example, there was a period when orthopaedic surgeons always wore their collars turned up!

This can cause difficulties when giving staff support, as such an identity creates a cohesiveness within the group and they may feel others do not understand their particular pressures; therefore a level of trust has to be developed before external support can be given in a way that is acceptable and valued. Often a close knit camaraderie exists; it is even seen in areas such as midwifery and paediatrics where there are particularly strong professional identities distinguishing midwives, paediatric nurses and general nurses.

Ethical issues

There are some areas which have their own powerful ethical issues.

These can forge a very close-knit approach among the staff, for example those looking after HIV/AIDS patients, because the patients are judged by others for their lifestyle and there is a general fear of AIDS, all of which helps to create a 'tightly bonded missionary group'. Staff feel strongly that they have to protect the interests and confidentiality of clients, and they have a strong need to educate the world to appreciate their needs. There is a significant incidence of stress-related illness among those working in these fields (Miller 1995). In fact many staff only last for a short while in the job.

Confidentiality can prove an area of conflict for staff working in any area similar to AIDS, and particularly for any member of staff concerned with counselling or similar support activities. It is important to provide independent supervision and support for staff in this position.

Some ethical issues are more dramatic than others in the minds of the public and the media and arouse great public concern, which causes much stress. These fall into two main groups:

(1) Perpetual issues concerning life itself and the quality of life, including ethical issues about patients who refuse treatment (e.g. Jehovah's Witnesses) and controversial discussion over treatment such as disconnecting life support systems.

(2) Areas where staff work on the frontiers of medicine and are concerned with issues such as IVF trials or the use of untried techniques and experimental research. They are exposed to a body of opinion expressing loud disagreement over something which has never happened before. Every movement of the frontiers of knowledge is a challenge to those who hold static beliefs. The difficulties become apparent when the media picks on these polarised views to create a debate.

With hindsight today's ethical dilemma often appears of less importance when seen in the general context of progress or in the light of new knowledge. It is interesting to note that in their infancy, surgery, anaesthetics and organ transplants were opposed by significant numbers as being unethical. Indeed at times all were described as being the 'work of the devil'.

In such an important area there is a need to create a supportive environment and to ensure that there are occasions when staff can question and analyse the situation with other people involved and can feel valued, supported and cared for.

Conflicting values

This moves into the whole area of conflict of values and personal beliefs, because it is threatening for those who find it difficult to accept change, to find that their beliefs are challenged. There is a conscience clause for staff who wish to opt out of certain procedures but this does not solve the problem because there are no 'opt out' clauses for caring for the patient. So staff have to continue to give care where the treatment procedures may be against their principles.

Dilemmas occur, for example, where doctors may refuse a patient heart surgery when they continue to smoke heavily. The decision might involve making treatment available for another patient who has a higher chance of a successful outcome and who might otherwise be deprived of that cure; but on the other side there is the commitment to treat fairly and without discrimination on any basis, including colour, race culture or judgement of lifestyle. Prioritising decisions can be painful ones.

Controversial areas exist where people are faced with courses of action which they find difficult to equate with their beliefs. For example, a gynaecologist who is not willing to carry out abortions would be unlikely to be appointed to a consultancy post these days.

Questioning practices involves not only the process of reasoning but also one's beliefs, therefore it engages the whole person. It is important to allow a high level of debate, giving information so that the facts can be assessed on all sides. This must be followed by support allowing for both reason and belief, and this involves supporting the person in the moral and personal dilemmas they are facing.

Those with fundamentalist beliefs find themselves in difficulties. They are placed into an impossible conflict with important parts of their own support networks, particularly for specific religious groups. They may find their long held beliefs and values undermined, which threatens them, creating the insecurity born of uncertainty. Their behaviour and professional care and practice may be criticised by their own friends and relatives where it is out of line with their religious beliefs and practices.

Ethics and values in the workplace

There are other values presenting particular difficulties in the modern, highly pressurised demands of business practices, in the intensity of work required in technology and pharmacology, in the need for constant assessment and reassessment or for instant or rapid decision taking which leads to actions with long reaching consequences. For example, there are pressures of this kind in A&E or in operating departments and to some degree in most other areas, particularly where there is a need to be constantly functioning at a highly intellectual and analytical level. There are demanding levels of work in which support is essential and where the person often needs time out for reflection and reassessment. Doctors, for example, get study leave or conference time which is less available to many practical nurses and paramedics. Life is more demanding on junior doctors where they have less access to time out.

Negative aspects

There are many unpopular decisions which have to be taken, such as closing beds or wards when resources are restricted, with some procedures suspended in order to maintain minimal standards for care and treatment. Cold surgery is one example where these difficult decisions have to be made with untold suffering to the patient. Staff know these decisions are causing suffering and need special support at these times.

> A surgeon was heard to say that with advances made in his field of work he could work at a reasonable level for six months, and then would have exhausted his budget and so could take six months off. This was particularly frustrating as the skills and technical resources were available, but not the money. The greatest stressor was knowing people who could be treated would inevitably die before reaching the operating table.

Many surgeons tend to opt out because they cannot sustain these pressures long term. So this is an important area to examine because individuals who know they have the ability to do something creative in the relief of suffering and are prevented from doing it, find this a powerful stressor. Also the effect of such restrictions on their own efficiency level is evident.

Stress for managers

Frequently conflict arises for managers in areas of resource allocation, particularly when working with clinicians all of whom are clamouring for resources. Medical knowledge has increased but managers seeking to provide a total service find themselves in difficult circumstances with conflicts between a range of clinicians when they know resources are not adequate. It is difficult for managers to know what to do, as they see the needs and hear the demands but find they cannot fulfil their responsibilities in a way which satisfies the clinicians or their own standards of care.

Attitudes in the workplace

Mental health is an example of a difficult specialist area which throws up many issues related to ethics and attitudes. There are difficulties relating to sectioning, to the right to give consent and to how far it is right to go on giving treatment without the patient's consent. This presents staff with much difficulty and conflict. There are many difficulties relating to early discharge and community care, where people are being discharged before staff feel they are ready to go out. Because of the lack of resources there is a lack of support to patients in the community and indeed this creates problems with lack of support for community staff. This is all against the background of a depressing round of media criticism about treatment on discharge and failure to keep an eye on patients to notice any factors which would suggest a need for re-admission.

Another dilemma occurs in estimating how far freedom of the individual should be protected at the expense of others. The question is, where does the balance change with the need to protect the public, and from what does the public need protecting? Physical violence to staff and to the public has been widely debated, particularly where those released from more secure units, for example, rape or kill, creating public outcry with condemnation of those responsible for the release.

Another problem group are those who are verbally violent and have behaviour problems outside the home. At what point does this need treatment and that person need to be taken out of community care and back into hospital? The risk is of the clients coming into conflict with the law and moving into the criminal justice system, which in turn raises the question of whether this is the right place for them; indeed, is the law able to deal adequately with them? The number of people with psychiatric problems who are serving prison sentences is an ethical problem in itself. It is clearly a stressor for many working in the field of mental health and in the prison service.

Another factor is the question of feeling unsupported and undervalued, which can lead to high levels of frustration and sickness. The shorter the fuse the less understanding there is, and the more likely it is that situations with clients may become explosive.

> 'How could I sail alone on a stormy sea,
> with a broken mast and sails torn,
> without looking for someone to help me repair my ship,
> and continue the voyage with me.'

Michel Quoist: *The Breath of Love*

Yet another dimension in mental health is where relatives find it hard to accept that there is a mental health problem with a patient. Some become angry and the health care staff catch the brunt of this. It is also difficult for mental health workers to carry out a programme of care in the community where the community does not accept it (NIMBY: Not In My Back Yard, or not in my street, nor in our group). The difficulty in carrying out the programme called 'care in the community' is that it almost amounts to care 'imposed into the community'. In quite a few communities, a psychological wall is erected around a house accommodating a centre or clinic for those needing mental health care and thus it becomes another institution. There is much work to be done to try to bring together community mental health care workers, their clients and the community.

There is a strong need for support mechanisms in this field, and the recognition that care in the community is more demanding on resources and skilled staff than in-patient care. Other pressures arise for mental health workers when they know that, given more time, support and counselling, a person could live more effectively in the community. This care cannot be given because of heavy case loads and lack of time to concentrate on a particular patient.

Mix and match

This whole area of ethics, attitudes, values and beliefs presents a group of concerns which can generate uncertainties and pressures, and give rise to anxiety and threatening situations. It requires particular consideration for staff support provision. The aspects to consider are:

- Recognition of areas of potential difficulty
- Attempting to foresee and prevent or limit pressures and difficulties that might arise

- Providing special support within those areas; this may sometimes require a facilitator with special skills, knowledge and experience in the issues concerned
- Recognising where staff may find particular personal pressures and taking action to ameliorate these.

These provisions need to be built into any staff support system as an integral part of the system. The skill lies in getting the right mix or balance between recognition of need, prevention, and support services provided, and matching these with the resources available. Attitudes and values are important ingredients in establishing a philosophy of care, and so they can be the origins of considerable pressures where they are in conflict with each other. Some conflict will be inevitable in such contentious areas and where agonising decisions must be faced, so it needs to be balanced by effective and well targeted support mechanisms.

Key points

(1) Attitudes and values are basic ingredients for a caring philosophy, but they can also give rise to conflicts and pressures.
(2) Ethical considerations involve issues such as rights and responsibilities and confidentiality.
(3) Mental health care provides many examples of ways in which conflicts can arise.

Exercise

(11.1) Identify some ethical issues which cause considerable conflict for you in practical care situations. Why does conflict arise?
(11.2) What kind of support would help you to deal with some of the pressures caused in these situations?

Chapter 12

The Dynamics of Change – Culture and Creativity

Social life is characterised by universal attributes such as activity and constant movement. But change is more than this, the motion involves alteration and re-arrangement of some attributes. Smith (1976) points out that change is not true unless a *new pattern* has been formed as a result of these movements over time and in space, or a pattern emerges in another form.

Change is threatening to many, but it can be challenging to those who welcome an opportunity to be creative. Kelly (1989) considers conflict a necessary element in change, and where there are conflict and threat, frustration, stress and anxiety are generated. There may be conflict between individuals, between hierarchical groups, and within structural areas within organisations. Conflict may arise as roles change, and it may occur between groups. An organisation where there is no change and conflict can be stagnant, so a certain amount of change in life is essential and can be creative (Glen 1975).

Effects of change

Change and conflict can generate pressures for some or stimulate creativity for others, but either way they are always present in a dynamic situation. Change is an origin of pressure which needs recognition, and therefore needs an identifiable support provision.

Change can be 'active' when it occurs as a result of innovation or intervention from within the system, or 'passive' when it comes as the result of external influences, particularly cultural ones. Either way it is more than just movement; it involves permanent changes in *patterns* within the system or between units (Smith 1976).

Change has always happened, but the difference now is that the *pace* of change has speeded up considerably in the last 50 years or so. According to Toffler's predictions made in 1971, failure to adapt to change is a recipe for annihilation and leads to total breakdown and what he calls 'future shock' (Toffler 1971). The importance of these predictions is now apparent in all walks of life, as the effects of the increasing pace of change are seen. Its effects extend to changes in family life, in organisational and management structures, in business life and in technological growth, and can have penetrating effects on culture, beliefs and values, and roles within organisations. Toffler (1971) maintains that the battle to prevent future shock starts on a personal level. Blind acceptance or resistance to change do not work. What is needed is a selection of creative strategies, as options, strategies for re-shaping, deflecting, accelerating or decelerating change. He suggests that the remedy lies in having a range of strategies or options available, then being prepared to diagnose the need and put the appropriate strategy into operation. Disintegration can be avoided and many of the associated pressures can be diminished in this creative approach. Inevitably there are profound implications for health care services, as staff feel threatened by changes in job specifications, management styles and technological and scientific knowledge. Profound changes in value systems and beliefs can undermine the stability of groups and make individuals feel particularly insecure as they cannot keep up or adapt quickly enough, and feel overpowered as they are carried along by events.

Change is widely cited as a major cause of pressure in health care, but while structural changes are often blamed for their unsettling effects, sometimes there are deeper influences on the *value systems*. The overall influences of a changing culture are less well recognised, but can be more profound. Even the Greek philosophers say change is a constant element and a basic characteristic of life:

> 'Everything flows,' said Heraclitus, 'everything is in constant flow and movement, nothing is abiding. Therefore we cannot step twice into the same river, when I step into the river for the second time, neither I nor the river are the same.'

> Heraclitus, quoted by Gaarder (1995)

Cultural influences

Any staff support system needs to be flexible and adaptable in order to respond to rapid change, and to take note of cultural influences which are the 'fabric' or 'glue' holding the wider society together, providing cohesiveness. Attention is focused frequently on the structure of organisations, without realising how important the culture is, as this is less tangible. Culture affects whole societies and civilisations, as well as particular organisations which can cultivate their own aspects of a caring culture (Oakley 1995).

So the health care worker is influenced by the culture of the world at large and society in general. The wider culture affects both the culture of the organisation and the lifestyle and attitudes of the individual; also the way the individual relates to the organisation.

The health services were 'born with a culture grounded in concepts of social welfare' (Oakley 1995), and now the prevailing culture comes from a world where managers and administrators are to the fore, rather than professionals. Services are led by financial accountability, budgets, productivity, purchasers and providers within a business ethos. Clearly there are potential conflicts within the system, not least those which bring changes in long held values. The conflicts occur between the ideals and beliefs which motivate many professionals who enter the health care fields, and the current business culture created by government.

> An article in September 1996 (Lilley 1996) opened with the title 'Strategic management is a waste of time'. Roy Lilley of Nottingham University told health service managers, 'management is finished and strategy no longer works'. He went on to say that five year strategies and three year programmes were pointless as no one can predict the future with any confidence. 'Tactics and techniques,' he said, 'are now essential...'

Structures and strategies are important to shape our thinking and give a sense of purpose, but in practice the key words are *flexibility and adaptability*, two qualities good managers and staff selectors will be seeking.

Conflict and change – some current realities

Concept of fairness

One ethical principle predominant in today's culture is *fairness*. There are two aspects of fairness to consider:

(1) Fairness within an organisation relating to groups, departments and professions
(2) Fairness within the organisation as related to the outside world.

One pertinent example is pay. This has considerable effects on staff morale giving rise to conflicts. In 1996 nurses were offered a 2% pay rise topped up by local pay from within each trust, while doctors in the same trust were given 6.5%. In the world outside, MPs received a 26% increase while the rates of increase for directors or board members of companies on bonus schemes were as high as 180% of salary. The comparison is emphasised by the different starting points for these increases. The saying goes, '3% of peanuts is peanuts'.

This element of 'fairness' can be seen as a reflection of how both government and society value the caring professions. Another aspect of fairness is the inequality of basic facilities within which staff operate. Facilities in banks, building societies, shops etc. appear luxurious compared with the accommodation provided for health care staff. Similarly, the decor and facilities in management areas show considerable differences from those in other places.

Professional ideologies, prevailing cultures and political dilemmas

A conflict exists for staff who have ideals and beliefs which produce a strong motivation to serve the needs of the sick and suffering to the highest standards of care, and for the largest number. They find themselves working against constraints of budgeting and managing which they perceive as reducing the amount of time and resources available for direct delivery of that service.

Another area causing confusion and conflict is where values and beliefs are in conflict with a prevailing culture from the political arena. The individual can feel pulled between the desire to serve patients and the need to maintain decent living standards to care for their families. Many staff have young families to provide for and need their pay to be sufficient to prevent constant worry. This worry is a stressor which has a powerful negative effect on the ability to care for others. To feel underpaid in relation to other groups within the service, and in relation to other groups outside, is often interpreted as not being valued by government and society.

Legal issues

Litigation is another area where cultural attitudes are changing considerably, with far reaching effects on health care. The general public are now much more knowledgeable and aware, partly through the media, and expect their rights to be safeguarded. Surgeons in some countries are becoming extremely wary of working in contentious areas because of the likelihood of litigation if the outcome is not successful. Litigation in this country is becoming a serious threat.

Similarly staff are becoming more aware of their rights in relation to their employer's duty to recognise staff needs, particularly in areas where the pressures are excessive.

> 'Legislation found in Section 2(1) of the Health and Safety at Work Act 1974 places a duty on every employer to ensure … the health, safety and welfare at work of all his employees. Regulation 3 of the Management of Health and Safety at Work Regulations 1992 requires every employer to make a suitable and sufficient assessment of the risks to the health and safety of his employees to which they are exposed while at work so that he can take appropriate and preventive and protective measures.'
>
> MSF Guide (1995)

This legislation is extended to cover both physical and mental health risks, which emphasises the importance for managers to provide a good staff support system.

Transcultural issues

Another factor which affects the provision of support care for staff and patients and is constantly undergoing change, is that of transcultural understanding and care. Multicultural and multifaith issues have been nominally on the health care agenda for some years, with very little evidence of any real development of understanding of the cultures and wide ranging issues concerned, apart from observations about certain practices. With the growing confidence of ethnic groups to articulate their needs and voice their dissatisfaction with deficiencies, they have been able to make these more known and seek responses.

A more committed response has been demanded by government and the Department of Health, primarily through the Patients' Charter. This has drawn attention to the real issues of understanding the complexities of cultural needs, highlighting the importance of attitudes and the staff training needed. To care effectively in a transcultural setting demands open attitudes and a willingness to value other cultures and beliefs as much as one's own. This can make heavy personal demands and put added responsibility on health care teams who are already very stretched.

Staff come into the caring professions from multicultural backgrounds and their needs also require recognition. Failure in understanding can generate conflict and pressure for all concerned, especially where individuals feel threatened by apparent discriminatory practices or opportunities. Appropriate staff support is essential in all these situations.

Conflicts of values and practicalities

One further example of an area of deficiency is where staff training is inadequate to equip staff for keeping up with the changes in technology and professional advances related to their job. Developments, particularly where there is a fast moving technological advance without proper training, can lead to lack of confidence and feelings of inadequacy with a fear of making mistakes. This is a powerful stressor.

Underlying most of these issues is the fact that staff need to learn to care for themselves as they care for patients. At times this attitude can lead to personal conflicts and conflicts with employers, especially when there is an imbalance of demands and resources. This emphasises the importance of appointing staff who can adapt to change. It means offering in-service training to maintain confidence levels. Managerial staff need to be alive to potential areas of conflict and prevailing cultural attitudes, both within and outside the organisation.

These examples illustrate the importance of recognising the influence of the wider culture in establishing staff support systems. They also emphasise that if systems are to function smoothly they need to take into account cultural patterns and the process of change, to be ready with alternatives, and to be able to adapt and respond to changing conditions.

This quotation from Handy is a useful reminder that organisations need structures and systems but they are made up of people and not just pairs of hands or role occupants:

'Organisations used to be perceived as gigantic pieces of engineering with largely interchangeable human parts. We talked of structures and systems, of inputs and outputs, of control devices and managing them...'

'Today the language is not that of engineering but of politics with talk of cultures and networks, teams and coalitions, influence and power rather than control, of leadership not management.'

Handy (1995)

We are now ready to move into the final section of the book, bringing together the main concerns looked at to present a comprehensive, integrated approach to staff support systems.

Key points

(1) Change is a constant factor in all areas of life and progress.
(2) It is always with us and can be a source of threat and conflict or creativity.
(3) Some of the effects of change on health care staff relate to growing awareness of legal aspects, litigation and ethnic minorities.
(4) These issues need a special approach to staff care.

Exercises

(12.1) Outline some of the changes taking place in your workplace at this time. What effects are they having on the staff?
(12.2) Discuss how these changes can be approached to ensure a creative outcome.

Section V

The Support Process Through Change and Adaptation

Chapter 13

Putting it All Together – Integration and Involvement

> 'We had the experience but missed the meaning,
> And approach to the meaning restores the experience
> In a different form...
> ...the past experience revived in the meaning
> Is not the experience of one life only
> But of many generations.'
>
> T.S. Eliot: *The Dry Salvages*

The creation of a beautiful tapestry will bring together a blend of patterns, colours, shapes and materials, but the creator knows that if it is to remain functional and serve its purpose effectively over a period of time, the fabric which is the foundation for the creation is a most important element. The finished product will be enhanced if it brings together a blend of different skills and ideas, which work together to form a work of art.

A book like this one draws its inspiration from two main sources:

(1) Research findings and factual reports over the years and from current projects
(2) Experience both from personal 'hands on' practice and shared experience with colleagues.

This is particularly evident when considering the development of staff support in health care. Some early research studies were from Menzies' work on defence against anxiety in health care staff (Menzies 1960b), Revans work on relationships between staff morale and patient recovery (Revans 1962) and Birch's study on nurse wastage (Birch 1975).

The report of the committee on nursing (Department of Health 1972) made a strong plea for personal counselling for nurses, and two major teaching hospitals reported on their pioneering efforts (Owen

151

1993). This review draws attention to the growing interest in the 1970s and 1980s in defining stress, its nature and causes and its damaging effects on individuals. Little evidence existed on the value of intervention methods; those recorded related mainly to counselling services, support groups and crisis intervention. From 1985 onwards focus began to develop on management and organisational aspects of stress.

These trends were supported by Cartwright (1996). Chapter 5 of this book describes how studies have moved through consideration of positive and negative effects of stress, the economic and personal costs of unmanaged stress and the benefits of having a healthy workforce. Studies reveal the importance of primary, secondary and tertiary prevention and participation between employers and employees in the involvement of promoting a healthy workforce and environment (Cartwright 1996). This full circle approach has also been evident from many reports of practical experience which relate to local initiatives and innovative interventions.

It is interesting that research is supporting much of the practical observation made by practitioners. This underlines the value of seeing the picture as a whole and recognising the many 'fibres' that need to be woven into the fabric to produce the tapestry described in the opening of this chapter.

Process of staff support as presented in this book

In this book the reader will have undertaken a journey. Section II looks at the different theories on the nature and origins of various pressures of health care staff. The journey then moved through a range of different perspectives and the different responses from individuals concerned.

This is the background 'map' to accompany the 'guide book' aspects of Section III on practical interventions to bring support to individuals through team and organisational support. Section IV broadens the vision to take in the wider world and cultural influences. The reader is now ready to bring all these aspects together into the whole picture, and to see what holds the tapestry together.

The figures in Chapters 2 and 3 are two dimensional, but in real life the picture is never static as the structure exists in the context of constant change. All the parts move in relation to each other, which means the framework may no longer be right for all situations.

Cultural aspects

The importance of cultural influences, as seen in Chapter 12, is becoming more widely recognised in the approach to staff support. The two main aspects to take into account, which have emerged in Section IV, relate to:

- The internal culture of the organisation
- The external culture of the outside world.

Figure 13.1 shows the relationship between these two as the whole picture becomes clear.

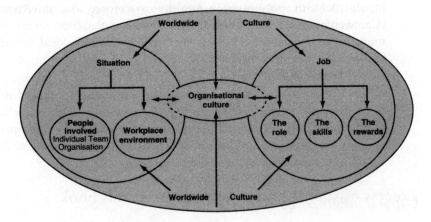

Fig. 13.1 Integrated model of the internal culture of the organisation and the external culture of the outside world.

Internal culture of an organisation

The internal culture of an organisation reflects the culture of the wider world and responds to changes from within the organisation. Sometimes these two aspects may conflict and sometimes they may harmonise. The internal culture can, however, be influenced by the people involved, the philosophy of care established within the workplace and the organisational structure.

'The organisational culture concerns symbols, values, ideologies and assumptions which operate ... to guide and fashion individual and business behaviour. It has been defined as simply "the way in which things get done within the organisation" ... It functions to create cohesiveness and maintain order and regularity in the lives of its members.'

Cartwright & Cooper (1994)

The culture is reflected in management styles and staff relationships, and also in the nature and quality of staff support.

The external culture

Organisational life will be affected by many aspects of the external culture, including attitudes to work, government policies, current knowledge and the nature of technological change. The nature and pace of change in the wider world will influence internal mechanisms. Figure 13.1 shows the relationships between these cultural influences, in particular:

- The way in which the *internal* culture of an organisation pervades all aspects of its structure
- The underlying 'fabric' that holds together the relationships between the various parts
- The way in which the *external* culture can also influence the various parts and relationships looked at in the course of this book, and can affect the functioning processes.

Cultural influences on staff support

Figure 3.1 sets out different elements of organisational and human life to be addressed during the process of creating a good staff support system. Like the tapestry, they will need not only a framework or overall pattern within which the elements function, but an overall fabric which holds them together. In the case of staff support, the culture is the critical fabric within which any organisation, team or individual operates. It is the culture which helps to mould those who come into it, to acquire what might be called the 'corporate identity'. It is the feature which distinguishes an organisation, making it stand out from others and enhancing performance. This is why in industry or the armed forces a heavy emphasis is placed upon a cohesive culture.

This is seen in Japanese culture where health is highly regarded in industry. It is shown in the emphasis on physical training, in which all staff from the most senior to the most junior participate daily. The provision of facilities for fitness training and leisure activities is seen as part of encouraging individuals to take responsibility for their own health within their team and organisation. This trend is an indication of the value placed on the individual and team and is reflected in performance and output. It encourages staff at all levels, as part of the team, to 'own' the aims of the whole organisation. It generates a real pride in the work in which they are engaged.

> This approach was echoed in the USA in an aircraft firm where a team of 5000 staff was brought in to work on a new plane. The value placed on each individual through the corporate identity was demonstrated through a corporate approach and established through daily meetings. All staff had a chance to feed in ideas about progress and ways of working. Ultimately production was so efficient that a plane was ready for testing well in advance of schedule, something quite unheard of previously in the industry. It was also noted that absenteeism and sickness rates were exceptionally low.

An open culture allows the identification of pressures and needs, which leads to an integrated approach to staff support. One of the most powerful external cultural influences is the effect of change. It may mean frameworks within the organisation have to change if they are not right for the current situation. Examples of external influences in the form of structural or attitudinal change are:

- Limits imposed by financial restrictions and resources available
- Marked differences in kinds of materials and equipment needed, leading to changing allocation of resources
- Practices which are speeding up and becoming either less or more labour intensive
- New technology which may require more complex controls or new operating skills
- Changes in skills required and new knowledge implications.

The speed with which these changes are imposed will pose a threat to staff, with consequent pressures. The staff support framework needs to take account of these uncertainties if provision is to be made to target priority areas. *Adaptation* and *flexibility* therefore remain two essential qualities, both for individuals and for the organisational framework. There are, however, some 'constants' in the situation:

- *Change will occur* and cannot be prevented or resisted in the long term, so preparation is essential

- The *principles* involved in staff support do not change and can remain as guidelines however much the framework must adapt
- Staff always need to be valued and to contribute to decision making in such a way that their creative potential can be fully realised and they can 'own' the work.

One of the greatest threats to staff is that of being unable to maintain the standards of care demanded by their professional commitment and the aspirations which they held when entering the health care services.

Achievement – the reality of a caring culture

There are no simple answers and no short cuts to creating staff support systems. Changes may not occur overnight but the first step is to put the process in motion in the context of the whole picture presented in Fig. 13.1. Once this overall vision has been understood and accepted by the whole team, it is possible for everyone to move forward, with individuals, teams and management working together. Some basic principles can be followed as guidelines, for example:

- Start wherever you are now
- Everyone has a contribution to make
- Assessment of the local situation and needs is important
- Use local evidence and draw on current research studies to support a proposal
- Assess existing resources and ensure they are used efficiently
- Decide on priorities to be dealt with immediately within the existing budget
- Develop a strategy for longer term planning
- Involve staff from all levels of the organisation in the process
- Keep the situation under constant review and be ready to adapt to changing needs.

Provision of staff support cannot be considered a luxury but must be an integral part of the organisational structure. It is part of the 'staple diet' in a caring environment and is basic to the delivery of good patient care. The responsibility for this caring environment belongs to everyone in the health care services. Managers and all staff are involved in the evolutionary process of creating and maintaining appropriate mechanisms, services and care for both colleagues and patients.

It is this process which empowers individuals to care for themselves, team members to care for each other and managers to ensure the organisation values its staff by the creation of a safe, healthy and responsive organisational structure and working environment.

'If each note of music were to say: one note does not make a symphony,
   there would be no symphony.
If each word were to say: one word does not make a book,
   there would be no book.
If each brick were to say: one brick does not make a wall,
   there would be no house.
If each drop of water were to say: one drop does not make an ocean,
   there would be no ocean.
If each seed were to say: one grain does not make a field,
   there would be no harvest.
If each one of us were to say: one act of love cannot save mankind,
   there would never be peace and justice on earth.
... Begin now! Why are you waiting'

Michel Quoist: The Breath of Love

References

Albrecht, T.L. & Adelman, M.B. (1984) Social support and life stress. *New Directions for Human Communications Research*, 11, 3–32.

Alexander, D.A. (1993) Staff support groups: do they support and are they even groups? *Palliative Care*, 7, 127–32.

Alexander, D.A., Walker, L.G., Innes, G. & Irving, B. (1993) *Police Stress at Work*. The Police Foundation, London, in association with the Department of Mental Health, University of Aberdeen.

Aurelio, J.M. (1993) An organisational culture that optimizes stress; acceptable stress in nursing. *Nursing Admin. Quarterly*, 18(1) 1–10.

Bach, R. (1972) *Jonathan Livingston Seagull*. Pan Books Ltd., London.

Bayntum-Lees, D. (1992) Reviewing the nurse patient partnership. *Nursing Standard*, 6(42) 36–9.

Biley, F.C. (1989) Stress in high dependency units. *Intensive Care Nursing*, 5, 134–41.

Bilie, D. (1993) Road to recovery, post-traumatic stress disorder: the hidden victim. *Journal of Psychological Nursing*, 31, 9.

Birch, J. (1975) *To Nurse or Not to Nurse*. Research Series. Royal College of Nursing, London.

BMA (1993) *The Morbidity and Mortality of the Medical Profession*. British Medical Association, London.

Booth, C. (1995) *Helping Patients with Cancer*. PhD Thesis. *NASS Newslink*, June 1995.

Borrill, C., Hayes, C. & Carter, A. (1996) NHS Workforce Initiative Phase 1. Obtainable from Institute of Work Psychology, University of Sheffield.

Bradshaw, W.J. (1972) The concept of social need. *New Society*, 30, 640–43.

Carlisle, C., Baker, G.A., Riley, M. & Dewey, M. (1994) Stress in midwifery: a comparison of nurses and midwives. *Advanced Journal of Nursing Studies*, 31(1) 13–22.

Cartwright, S. (1996) *Managing Pressures, Responding Creatively*. Unpublished paper given at NASS Conference, October 1996.

Cartwright, S. & Cooper, C. (1994) *No Hassle! Taking the Stress Out of Work*. Century Business Ltd, London.

Channon, M., Long, J. & Stoter, D. (1990) *Support Systems in the Health Care Settings*. NASS Occasional Paper No. 4. National Association for Staff Support, Woking.

Charlton, B.G. (1992) Stress. *Journal of Medical Ethics*, 18, 156–9.

Cooper, C. (1988) Hotline team helps doctors enslaved by sickness trap. *Hospital Doctor*, 68(16).

Cooper, C. (1995) *Handbook of Stress, Medicine and Health*. CRC Press, Florida.

Cooper, C. & Smith, M.J. (1986) *Job Stress and Blue Collar Work*. Wiley & Sons, Chichester.

Cooper, C., Cooper, R.E. & Eaker, L.H. (1988) *Living with Stress*. Penguin Books, London.

Cooper, C., Sadri, G., Alison, T. & Reynolds, P. (1990) Stress counselling in the Post Office (research). *Counselling Psychology Quarterly*, 3(1) 3–11.

Cooper, C., Luikkonen, P. & Cartwright, S. (1996) *Stress Prevention in the Workplace: Assessing the Costs and Benefits to Organisations*. European Foundation for the Improvement of Living and Working Conditions, Loughlinstown, Dublin.

Cox, T. (1978) *Stress*. University Park Press, Baltimore.

Cox, T. (1993) *Stress Research and Stress Management: Putting Theory to Work*. HSE Research Contract Report No.61/1993 with University of Nottingham. Obtainable from HSE Books, Sudbury, Suffolk.

Cox, T., Leather, P. & Cox, S. (1990) Stress, health and organisations. *Occupational Health Review*, Feb/March, 13–18.

Cushway, D. (1995) Understanding stress and coping. *British Journal of Therapy and Rehabilitation*, 2(1) 615–20.

Department of Health (1972) *Report of Committee on Nursing*. (The Briggs Report) Cmmd 5115. HMSO, London.

Dewe, P. (1991) Primary appraisal, secondary appraisal and coping: their role in stressful work encounters. *Journal of Occupational & Organisational Psychology*, 65, 81–8.

Downey, V., Bengiamin, M. Hever, L. & Juhl, N. (1995) Dying babies and associated stress in NICU. *Nurses Neonatal Network* ,14(1) 41–5.

Eliot, T.S. (1969) *Collected Poems 1909–1962*. Faber and Faber, London, and Harcourt Brace & Co., London.

Elkin, F. (1960) *The Child and Society*. Chapters 2 and 3. Raiden Hume, New York.

Farman, R. & Gore, G. (1995) Good intentions in NHS Trusts for staff support. *NASS Newslink*, September 1995.

Farrell, M. (1992) A process of mutual support, establishing a support network for nurses caring for dying patients. *Professional Nurse*, October, 10–13.

Foss, B.M. (1961) *Determinants of Infant Behaviour*, Vol. 1. Methuen, London.

Foss, B.M. (1963) *Determinants of Infant Behaviour*, Vol. 11. Methuen, London.

Frazer, G.H. & Sechrist, S.R. (1994) A comparison of occupational stressors in selected allied health disciplines. *Health Care Supervision*, 13(1) 81–9.

Gaarder, J. (1995) *Sophie's World*. Phoenix, London.

Glen, F. (1975) *The Social Psychology of Organisations*. Methuen, London.

Griffiths, A., Cox, T. & Barlow, C. (1996) Employer's responsibility, the assessment and control of work-related stress: a European perspective. *Health and Hygiene*, 17, 62–70.

Handy, C. (1991) *The Age of Unreason*. Arrow Business Books, London.

Handy, C. (1995) *The Gods of Management*. Arrow Business Books, London.

Harris, J.R. (1991) The utility of the transaction approach for occupational stress research. *Journal of Social Behaviour*, Handbook on Job Stress (special issue), 21–9.

Harvey, P. (1992) Staff support groups, are they necessary? *British Journal of Nursing*, 1(5) 256–8.

Hawthorne, J.W. (1932) Cited in *The Organisation Man* (1956) (White W.H.), pp37–40. Pelican Books, London.

Health at Work in the NHS (1995a) *Organisational Stress in the NHS*. OPUS Report, Health Education Authority, London.

Health at Work in the NHS (1995b) *Measuring and Monitoring Sickness Absence in the NHS*. Health Education Authority, London.

Health at Work in the NHS (1996) *Organisational Stress. Planning and Implementing a Programme to Address Organisational Stress in the National Health Service*. OPUS Report, Health Education Authority, London.

Hinds, P.S., Quarenen, T.I., Hickey, S.S. & Mangum, G.M. (1994) A comparison of stress response sequence in new and experimental paediatric/oncology nurses. *Cancer Nursing*, 17(1) 61–71.

Hingley, P. (1991) A stressful occupation. *Nursing Times*, 87(25) 63–6.

Hingley, P. & Marks, R. (1991) *The Costs of Stress and the Benefits of Stress Management*. NASS Occasional Paper No.5, National Association for Staff Support, Woking.

Hoff, B. (1982) *The Tao of Pooh*. Mandarin, London.

HSE (1990) *Mental Health at Work*. Medical Division, Health and Safety Executive, London.

IRS (1991) Employee Assistance Trends. IRS Survey of EAP Programmes. Industrial Relation Service, 18 Highbury Place, London.

Johnson, W. (1991) Predisposition to emotional stress and psychiatric illness amongst doctors: the role of unconscious and experimental factors. *British Journal of Medical Psychology*, 64, 317–29.

Jones, G. (1995) The Employer's Obligation in Relation to Staff Support. NASS Occasional Paper No.10. National Association for Staff Support, Woking.

Kellner-Pringle, M. (1975) *The Needs of Children*. Chapter 1. Hutchinson, London.

Kelly, J. (1989) *Organisational Behaviour*. Homewood Darsey.

Lazarus, R.S. & Folkman, S. (1984) *Stress, Appraisal, Coping*. McGraw Hill, New York.

Lilley, P. (1996) News report. *Nursing Standard*, 10, 52.

Manufacturing Science and Finance Guide (1995) *Preventing Stress at Work*. Safety information No.40. MSF Health and Safety Office, Bishop's Stortford.

Meekin, S. (1990) Post-traumatic stress counselling. *Nursing Standard*, 5(8) 32–4.

Menon, N. & Akhilesh, R.B. (1994) Functionally dependent stress among managers: a new perspective. *Journal of Managerial Psychology*, 9(3) 13–22.

Menzies, L. (1960a) A Case Study on the Functioning of Social Systems as a Defence against Anxiety in Human Relations. Tavistock, London.

Menzies, L. (1960b) Institutional defence against anxiety. *Human Relations*, 13, 95–121.

Meutz, C. (1995) Occupational health, dealing with stress. *Nursing Standard*, 10(2) 27–30.

Miller, D. (1995) Dying to Care? Occupational Morbidity and Burnout, and Preferences for Staff Support in HIV and Oncology Health Care. *Unpublished doctoral thesis*. University of Nottingham.

Montague, S. (1979) Paper at conference of Association of Integrated and Degree Courses, York. Unpublished conference report.

Moore, W. (1996) All stressed up and nowhere to go. *Health Service Journal*, September, 22–5.

Moss, R. (1995) Unpublished paper given at NASS conference April 1995.

NASS (1992a) *The Costs of Stress and Costs and Benefits of Stress Management*. Briefing Paper. National Association for Staff Support, Woking.

NASS (1992b) *A Charter for Staff Support*. National Association for Staff Support, Woking

Oakley, P. (1995) Cultural change within the NHS. *British Journal of Health Care Management*, 1(12).

O'Kell, S.P. (1993) Managing organisational stress, part I & part II. *Senior Nurse*, 13(3) 9–13, (4) 10–13.

Owen, G.M. (1988) For better, for worse: nursing in higher education. *Journal of Advanced Nursing*, 13, 1–11.

Owen, G.M. (1989) *A Study of the Marie Curie Community Nursing Service*. Marie Curie Memorial Foundation, London.

Owen, G.M. (1990) *Support Networks in Health Care*. NASS. Occasional Paper No.1, National Association for Staff Support, Woking.

Owen, G.M. (1993) *Taking the Strain. Stress Coping Mechanisms and Support Systems*. Literature Review, 5th Edition. National Association for Staff Support, Woking.

Payne, R. & Firth-Cozens, J. (1987) *Stress in Health Professionals*. Wiley, Chichester.

Quoist, M. (1992) *The Breath of Love*. Gill and Macmillan, Dublin.

Revans, R.W. (1962) Hospital attitudes and communication. *Sociological Review*, Monograph 5.

Revans, R.W. (1990) The hospital as a human system. *Behavioural Science*, 35.

Rogers, C. (1967) *On Becoming a Person*. Constable, London.

Rose, S. (1994) Counselling following trauma. *Counselling*, 5(2) 125–7.

Rose, S. (1995) Traumatic stress. A nure therapist role. *Nursing Standard*, 1, 31.

Rosenfeld, L.B. & Richman, J.M. (1987) *Stress Reduction for Hospice Workers: A Support Group Model in Stress and Burnout among providers*. The Hayworth Press.

Rosser, R. (1994) Post-traumatic stress disorder. *The Practitioner*, 238, 393–4, 396–7.

Rosser, R., Dewar, S. & Thompson, J. (1991) Psychological aftermath of Kings Cross Fire. *Journal of Royal Society of Medicine*, 84, 4–8.

Rutter, M. (1972) *Maternal Deprivation Re-assessed*. Penguin, London.

Schaffer, T. (1992) CPN stress and organisational change: a study. *Community Psychiatric Nursing*, Feb.

Scullion, R.A. (1994) An identification of stressors associated with accident and emergency departments and comparison of stress levels. *Accident and Emergency Nursing*, (2) 79–86.

Selye, H. (1950) *Stress*. Aita, Montreal.

Selye, H. (1960) *Stress in Health and Disease*. Butterworth, London.

Silverman, D. (1984) *The Theory of Organisations*. Heinemann Educational Books, London.

Sines, D. & Stoter, D.J. (1991) Creating a Caring Culture. NASS Occasional Paper No. 6. National Association for Staff Support, Woking.

Smith, A. (1976) *Social Change*. Longman Group, London and New York.

Spinks, P. & Bowering, P. (1990) Staff support. *Paediatric Nursing*, March, 19–20.

Storr, A. (1981) *The Integrity of the Personality*. Penguin, London.

Stoter, D.J. (1995a) *Spiritual Aspects of Health Care*, pp110. Mosby, London.

Stoter, D.J. (1995b) *Reflections on Response to Disaster Situations; Hindsight Brings New Perspectives to Preparation*. NASS Occasional Paper No. 9. National Association for Staff Support, Woking.

Thomas, R.S. (1984) *Later Poems 1972–1982*. Macmillan, London.

Toffler, A. (1971) *Future Shock*. Pan Books Ltd, London.

Traynor, M. & Wade, B. (1994) *The Morale of Nurses Working in the Community*. NHS Trust Service Report III, Daphne Heald Research Unit, Royal College of Nursing, London.

Tschudin, V. (1988) *Staff Support in Nursing Patients with Cancer. Why Nurses Need Support*. Prentice Hall, Hemel Hempstead.

Tschudin, V. (1992) *Ethics in Nursing*, 2nd ed. Butterworth & Heinemann, Oxford.

White, D. (1990) Health and stress: a self help guide. *Occupational Health Review*, 27, 11–14.

White, G. (1977) *Socialisation*. Social Processes Series. Longman, London and New York.

Woodham, A. (1995) *Beating Stress at Work*. Health Education Authority.

Further Reading

Alexander, D.A. (1991) Psychiatric intervention after Piper Alpha disaster. *Journal of the Royal Society of Medicine*, **84**, 8–11.

Alexander, D.A. (1992) Stress among palliative care matrons: a major problem for a minority group. *Palliative Medicine*, **6**, 111–24.

Beehr, T.A. & McGrath, J.E. (1992) Social support occupational stress and anxiety. *Anxiety, Stress & Coping*, **5**, 7–19.

BMA (1992) *Stress and the Medical Profession*. British Medical Association, London.

Cooper, C. (1996) Stress in the workplace. *British Journal of Hospital Medicine*, **55**(9) 559–63.

Cooper, C. & Sadri, G. (1990) Stress counselling at work. Counselling, *Journal of Sociological Behaviour and Personality*, **6**(7) 4, 11–23.

Cox, T. (1990) Stress management: palliative or preventive. *Occupational Health Review*, June/July, 202–4.

Elliott Binns, C. (1992) *Managing Stress in the Primary Care Team*. Blackwell Science, Oxford.

Gibson, M. (1991) *Order from Chaos: Responding to Traumatic Events*. Venture Press, Birmingham.

Grainger, C. (1994) *Stress Survival Guide*. British Medical Journal, London.

Owen, G.M. (1984) *The Role of Higher Education in Relation to Nursing Practice*. Paper given at Association of Integrated and Degree Courses in Nursing conference, July 1984.

Oxford Regional Health Authority (1993) *Workplace Health Promotion: a Review of Literature*. Directorate of Health Policy and Public Health, Oxford.

Roger, D. & Nash, P. (1995) A threat to health. *Nursing Times*, **91**(92).

Selye, H. (1976) *Stress in Health and Disease*. Butterworth, London.

Stapley, L. (1995) Cited in Health at Work in the NHS (1995a) – see references.

Stoter, D.J. (1990) Support Systems in Health Care Settings. Extracts from NASS Occasional Paper No. 4 by Channon, Long and Stoter. National Association for Staff Support, Woking.

Useful Addresses and Resources

British Association for Counselling
1 Regent Place
Rugby
Warwicks CV21 2PJ
Tel: 01788 550899/578328
BAC members are individuals and organisations concerned with counselling in a variety of settings. The information office publishes directories listing accredited counsellors.

British Holistic Medical Association (BHMA)
179 Gloucester Place
London NW1 6DX
Tel: 0171 262 5299
For all health staff interested in complementary therapies. Newsletters, meetings, books, conferences.

Child Bereavement Trust
Harleyford Estate
Henley Road
Marlow
Bucks SL7 2DX
Tel: 01628 488101
Provides support and counselling for bereaved families. Supplies videos, helpful literature and training for carers.

CRITEC – Crisis Counselling, Training, Education, Support, Information Service
Accident and Emergency
Leeds General Infirmary
Leeds LS1 3EX
Tel: 01132 2432799
CRITEC offers training, debriefing and an information service for those working with sudden death and other life crises.

Directory of Social Change
24 Stephenson Way
London NW1 2DP
Tel: 0171 209 5151
Useful short courses, mainly aimed at voluntary sector, including managing workloads, confident speaking, assertiveness, stress management, managing people.

Employee Advisory Resources Ltd (EAR)
Brunel Science Park
Kingston Lane
Uxbridge
Middlesex UB8 3PQ
Tel: 01895 271155
Workshops, journals and information on formal Employee Assistance Programmes (basically counselling). Provides EAP packages to employers.

Health Education Authority (HEA)
Health Promotion Information
Centre
Hamilton House
Mabledon Place
London WC1H 9TX
Tel: 0171 413 1994/5
Useful publications, and
information.

Health Pickup
NHS Training Directorate
St Bartholomew's Court
18 Christmas Street
Bristol BS1 5BT
Tel: 0117 291029
Open Learning specially designed
for health staff on topics including
stress management, teamwork, staff
development, change.

**Institute for Complementary
Medicine**
21 Portland Place
London WIN 3AF
This institute can supply names of
reliable practitioners of
complementary medicine such as
homeopathy, relaxation techniques
and osteopathy. It also has contact
with other support groups. Send
SAE for information, stating your
area of interest.

**International Stress Management
Association (ISMA)**
c/o The Priory Hospital
Priory Lane
London SW15 6JJ
Tel: 01256 21126
Journal, conferences, books, tapes,
videos, local support network,
research database, training.

**Jewish Bereavement Counselling
Service**
14 Chalgrove Gardens
London NW3 3PN
Tel: 0171 349 0839
Sends trained volunteer counsellors
to bereaved people. It operates in
Greater London, but can refer to
other projects and individuals
elsewhere.

The Lisa Sainsbury Foundation
8–10 Crown Hill
Croydon
Surrey
Tel: 0181 686 8808
This foundation offers information
and training support to those caring
for the dying and the bereaved.
Videos, literature and trainers can be
made available to organisations.

National Association for Staff Support (NASS)
9 Caradon Close
Woking
Surrey GU21 3DU
Tel: 01483 771599
Association of professionals with a common interest in co-ordinating and developing staff support resources for all health care staff. Produces its own literature, quarterly newsletter and organises conferences and workshops.

National Association for Widows (NAW)
c/o Stafford and District Voluntary Service Centre
Chell Road
Stafford ST16 2QA
Tel: 01785 45465
Advice, support and friendship is available to widows. This is a pressure group fighting against financial anomalies that widows have to face.

Nurseline
8–10 Crown Hill
Croydon
Surrey CR0 1RZ
Tel: 0181 681 4030
Advisory and 'signposting service' for nurses.

Relaxation for Living
29 Burwood Park Road
Walton on Thames
Surrey KT12 5LH
Tapes, books, training in relaxation.

Royal College of Nursing
20 Cavendish Square
London W1M 0AB
Tel: 0171 409 3333
Specialist services for members particularly library, legal and advisory.

Stillbirth and Neonatal Death Society (SANDS)
Argyle House
29–31 Euston Road
London NW1 2SD
Tel: 0171 833 2851
Offers advice and long-term support via local groups to newly bereaved parents of stillbirths and/or babies who die in their first months of life.

The Sue Ryder Foundation
Cavendish House
Sudbury
Suffolk CO10 8AY
Tel: 0178 280252
Six Sue Ryder homes in England specialise in cancer care. Visiting nurses care for patients in their own homes. Advice and bereavement counselling are provided.

Westminster Pastoral Foundation
23 Kensington Square
London W8 5HN
Tel: 0171 937 6956
Counselling services and education facilities for professional qualifications.

Additional resources

Preventing Stress at Work
An MSF Guide May 1995.
MSF Health and Safety Publication No. 40
MSF Health and Safety Office
Whitehall College
Dane O'Coys Road
Bishops Stortford
Herts CM23 2JN

Organisational Stress (Health at Work in the NHS)
Planning a programme to address organisational stress in the NHS
Hamilton House
Mabledon Place
London WC1H 9TX
Health Education Authority 1996

Staff Support in Health Care
An open learning package for anyone concerned with staff support
consisting of exercises, reading and self assessment. May be used by
individuals or for group work. Send S.A.E. to:

NASS (The National Association for Staff Support)
9 Caradon Close
Woking
Surrey GU21 3DU

Health at Work in the NHS
Resources directory for promoting health at work
Obtainable from the Health Education Authority (address as above).

NASS

NASS is a charitable association providing a networking and resource service for professionals who share an interest in promoting good staff support
practices for health care staff.

At the NASS central office, a database and literature resource provides a
national network of contacts and information for members and others.
NASS helps to co-ordinate local and national activities, and assists staff in
making the best of slender resources in their workplace. The organisation

aims to establish staff support on a national basis by supporting good management practices and promoting its Charter for Staff Support.

NASS offers its members:

- Assistance with setting up of local support systems.
- Information support through these local networks.
- Quarterly news on current trends in NEWSLINK, the NASS journal.
- A Charter for staff support, suitable for use by individuals and organisations.
- Discounts on NASS workshops, conferences and literature.
- Free copies of the NASS Manual and Charter.

For more information, please send an S.A.E. to:
The General Secretary
National Association for Staff Support
9 Caradon Close
Woking
Surrey GU21 3DU

Index